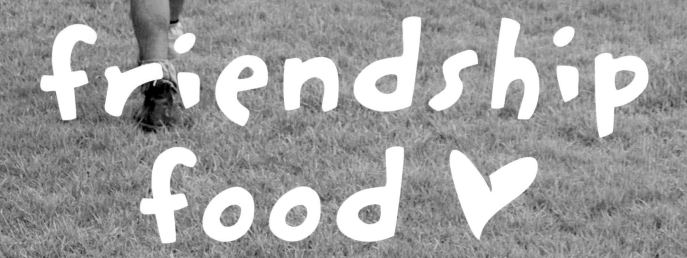

friendship food ♥

Delicious Feelgood Food

Free of Gluten, Yeast, Dairy, Egg and Refined Sugar

by Felicity Philp

with Julie Reardon, Kate Owen and Kylie Brasch

friendshipfood.com.au

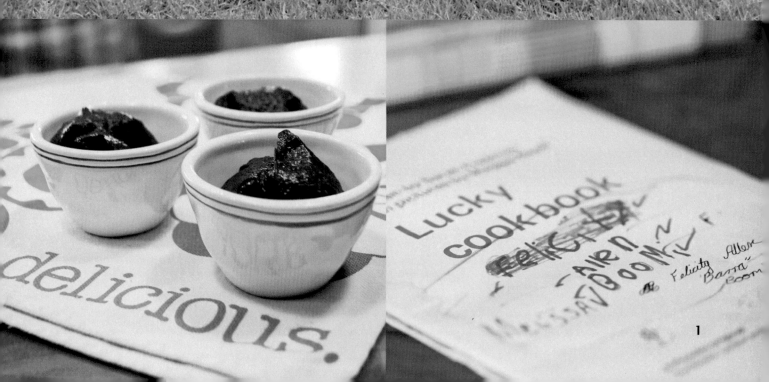

1

Dedicated to friends and families everywhere - may we create a bright, happy, healthy future together!

Thank you to our families for your love and support, especially during the process of creating this book, and for appearing in our photos!

Love Flick, Jules, Kate and Kylie

Credits:
Recipes and text © 2014 Felicity Philp
Layout, logo and graphic design © 2014 Julie Reardon
Photos on front cover and page 13 © 2014 Mandie O'Shea
Photos on page 9 and page 64 © 2014 Kate Owen
Photo on page 10 © 2014 Jennie Reardon
Photo on page 66 © 2014 Michael Owen
All other photos © 2014 Julie Reardon
Painting on page 2 © 2009 Mimi Philp
Cover makeup by Zazi Mineral Makeup (zazi.com.au).

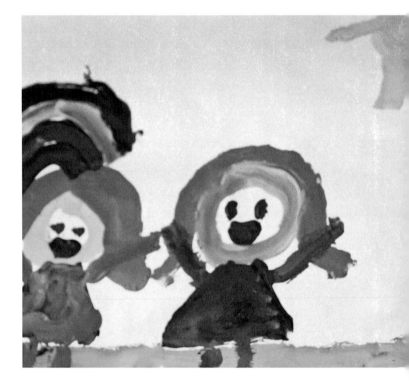

Balboa Press books may be ordered
through booksellers or by contacting:
Balboa Press
A Division of Hay House
1663 Liberty Drive
Bloomington, IN 47403
balboapress.com
1-(877) 407-4847

Because of the dynamic nature of the internet, any web addresses or links contained in this book may have changed since publication and may no longer be valid. The views expressed in this work are solely those of the author and do not necessarily reflect the views of the publisher, and the publisher hereby disclaims any responsibility for them.

ISBN: 978-1-4525-8431-7 (sc)
ISBN: 978-1-4525-8432-4 (e)

Library of Congress Control Number: 2013918509

Print information available on the last page.
Balboa Press rev. date 04/15/2015

Disclaimer:
We advise everyone to seek the opinion of a qualified medical practitioner before they make any changes to their diet. The stories, information and opinions documented in this book are used by the author to highlight the stages of her personal healing journey. They are not recommended as a personal healing method for anyone else and therefore should not be adopted as one's medicine to cure individual illness. There is no substitute for the advice of a qualified, medical practitioner. The author and the publisher will not accept any responsibility for any action or claim resulting from the use of information in this book.

Trademarks:
'Friendship Food™', 'Delicious Feelgood Food™', and 'Share Enjoy Nourish Thrive™' are all trademarks owned by Friendship Food Pty Ltd.

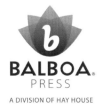

BALBOA
PRESS

A DIVISION OF HAY HOUSE

Welcome

Welcome to the start of an empowering friendship with food! The beginning of my friendship with food and the idea for this recipe book, came about five years ago after I experienced a flare-up associated with an autoimmune disorder I have. This prompted me to visit a natural healer who told me to take myself off gluten, yeast, dairy, eggs and refined sugar for three months. I remember driving home that day thinking 'what on earth am I going to eat?'

For me, eating well is not a hobby. I have to eat very, very well otherwise I am sick, sore and miserable.

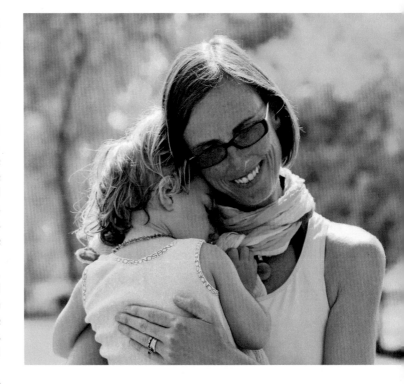

After visiting the healer, I set about converting recipes and researching ingredients and substitutes. I was amazed at the great food that was out there and all the healthy, tasty dishes that could be made without these key ingredients. My friends and family started asking me for recipes and details of where they could source the ingredients I was using. I soon realised many people knew someone who could benefit from my recipes.

Through my research of food and its origins, I have discovered an abundance of weird and wonderful ingredients, recipes and information about how food is best grown and prepared. The really wonderful thing is that this process continues to teach me how to be as healthy as I can be. I still love learning and trying out healthy food ideas!

In 2001 I was diagnosed with an autoimmune disorder called Scleroderma, which was also accompanied by some other unpleasant illnesses. My world fell apart momentarily as I desperately clung to quick-fix ideas and hunted down horrendously expensive magic pills that gave me relief while the placebo effect lasted.

My health was declining though and it continued to yo-yo up and down for some years until I went to see the healer who suggested eliminating certain foods from my diet. This advice has changed my life and I am so grateful I stuck with this eating strategy. The positive effects I felt were significant enough to kickstart me into making permanent changes to what I ate and what I fed my family.

The most profound difference since changing my diet has been that I now see the world through a very different window. I feel emotionally strong, I am very, very positive, I love life and I hope to make my mark on this world by helping others benefit from a better way of eating so that autoimmunity and other diseases do not plague our communities like they are threatening to right now.

Together with my gorgeous, very talented and outrageously supportive friends Kate Owen, Jules Reardon and Kylie Brasch, we have brought you 'Friendship Food', which is so much more than a recipe book. It is a kickstart to a more vibrant life. Just as it has done for me, the information in this book can provide you with a framework to create a more wonderful way of life. One that empowers you, making you question food and whether it is good enough for your precious body.

I am not a doctor, dietician or health practitioner.

I used to be a primary school teacher and now I am a Mum with an autoimmune disorder who changed her diet for three months and discovered a more natural way to alleviate the painful symptoms associated with her condition. By taking myself off gluten, dairy, yeast, eggs and refined sugar and substituting these ingredients for the best quality wholefoods I could afford, I felt fantastic. I was very relieved that there was hope for me out there and that it was tangible. I was also grateful that it didn't cost as much as miracle cures because at the time we were on one income with tiny children and excess money was scarce.

Even though I tout the benefits of natural remedies I still see the same medical specialist I first went to in 2001. I feel it is important to carry out the tests and take the medication she suggests. I do this because I have faith in her and I need her clinical advice. I am however, a great believer in complementary medicine and I am looking forward to seeing health practitioners of all modalities, working even more closely for the common good.

The information in this book is based on my own research and experiences whilst on my personal healing journey. Please consult a nutritionally trained and qualified health care professional before changing your diet and removing whole food groups from it. Whilst we wish you all the very best on your healthy eating journey, we cannot take responsibility for any adverse effects experienced by using the information and/or recipes in this book. The uniqueness of each and every one of our bodies and the vastly different lives we all lead, means every healing journey will be unique. We need to listen to our own bodies and be guided by them.

Being from a farming background, I'm sensitive to the fact that my food intolerances mean I can't personally continue to eat some foods produced by some farmers. The information I have put forward in this book is to let readers know how I have found relief by avoiding foods that exacerbate my Scleroderma symptoms. This information is not intended to impact farmers producing any of these foods.

I have written this book to share recipes and experiences with those wishing to learn more about practical, natural approaches to living with food intolerances and feeling great. I wish everyone who reads 'Friendship Food' a healthy, happy and delicious journey through life!

Felicity x

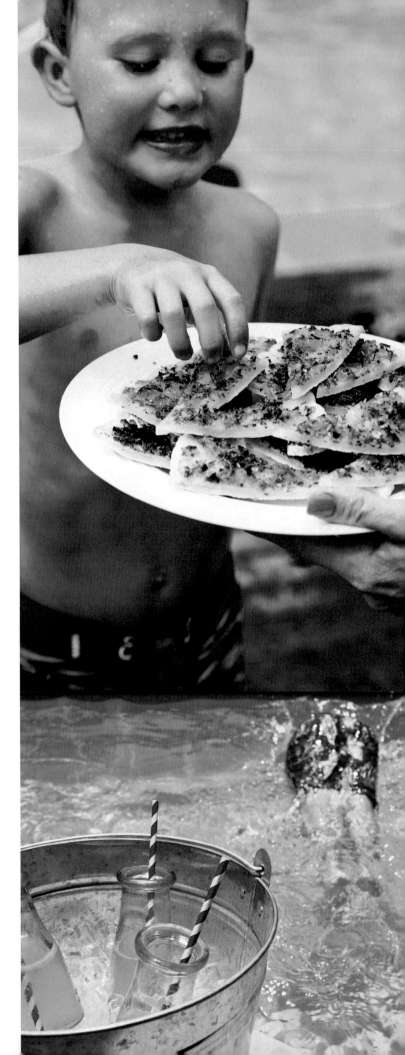

Contents

Welcome 3
Why Avoid Some Foods? 6
Global Health 8
Family & Community 10
My Healing Journey 12
Plan & Prep 15
Ingredients 16
Breakfast 20
   fruit platter 20
   bircher-style muesli 21
   plum porridge 21
   tomato zucchini salsa 22
   flick's baked beans 22
   potato hashies 23
   polenta coated bananas 23
Soups 24
   zesty carrot soup 24
   minty pea soup 24
   thai-style pumpkin soup 25
Salads & Light Meals 26
   cabbage noodle salad 26
   spiced beetroot 26
   chicken & veg stir-fry 27
   baby spinach & pumpkin salad 28
   easy rice salad 28
   quinoa, cranberry & chicken salad . . . 29
   rice paper rolls 29
Main Meals 30
   round deep dish lasagne 30
   cheese-free sprinkle 30
   rice noodle bolognese 31
   turkey tacos 31
   sweet beef curry 32
   chicken nuggets 33
   barra fish fingers 33
   orange, mustard & nut-glazed ham . . . 34
   miranda kerr's slow roasted chicken . . . 34
   mint & cranberry crusted lamb 35
Nibbles, Dips & Crackers 36
   salted & roasted nuts 36
   popcorn 36
   hommus 37
   helen's crispy seed crackers 38
   dukka 38
   carrot & coriander dip 39
   beetroot dip 39
   avocado & sweet chilli dip 39

Breads & Loaves 40
   farmer's fruit & nut loaf 40
   nutty cornbread 41
   teresa cutter's gluten-free bread . . . 41
   banana bread with orange spread . . . 42
   pizza dough & toppings 42-43
Cakes, Bars & Biscuits 44
   budgie snacks 44
   jam drops 45
   pecan puff bars 45
   rich spiced fruit cake 46
   carrot & apple cakes 47
   pear & almond biscuits 47
   honey joys 48
   choc walnut balls 48
   choc layer cake 49
Desserts & Sweet Treats 50
   chocolate coconut tart 50
   apple crumble 51
   almond custard 51
   chocolate mousse 52
   chocolate bark 52
   choc orange & easter egg truffles 53
   honey chocolate 53
   cashew, macadamia & raspberry tart . . . 54
   berry crumble 54
   mango ice blocks 55
   berry sorbet 55
Drinks 56
   watermelon slushies 56
   raspberry smoothies 56
   roseberry iced tea 57
   lemonade 57
Condiments 58
   onion jam 58
   raisin relish 58
   tomato sauce 59
   bbq sauce 59
   meat stock 59
   mayonnaise 59
   granny's gravy 59
   spicy orange dressing 60
   caper & dill sauce 60
   honey mustard dressing 60
Healthy Home 61
Food For Thought 62
Thank You 63
Index 64
References 66

Why Avoid Some Foods?

Allergy or intolerance?

If you have a food allergy then your body treats the offending food as an invading force and it reacts by emitting an immune response. This may be in the form of anaphylaxis, swelling or rashes. Alternatively, if you have a food intolerance this can mean the digestive tract is not functioning properly and symptoms can be felt immediately or over the course of hours, days, even weeks or months. When problem foods are eaten, the body produces more adrenalin to deal with these reactions, putting pressure on the immune system.

Why avoid gluten, eggs, dairy, yeast and refined sugar?

The following information gives a brief overview of each food type in question and the effect it may have on the body after it has been eaten.

Gluten

Gluten is a protein found in wheat, barley and rye. Problems with gluten arise when the body can't break down either the protein or the carbohydrates in the grains. Symptoms can include intestinal discomfort, bloating and wind. A more serious condition is Coeliac disease, an autoimmune disorder of the digestive tract, characterised by an inability to absorb nutrients from food.

Eggs

Problems with the consumption of eggs arise when there are insufficient enzymes in the small intestine to break down the proteins. Symptoms displayed in this case can affect the skin and respiratory system and cause post nasal drip, bloating, tummy cramps and diarrhoea.

Dairy

If you are intolerant to dairy products you may experience coughs, asthma, colds, sinus, skin problems, Irritable Bowel Syndrome, nausea, bloating and low iron levels. The trick with dairy intolerances is finding out which component of the dairy product is the issue. A qualified nutritional specialist can diagnose your symptoms to ascertain whether you may have an intolerance that is due to a problem digesting the protein (casein), the sugar (lactose), the fats (lipids) or alternatively if you are allergic to dairy products.

Yeast

Excess yeast from breads, baked sweets and alcohol can contribute to an overgrowth of fungal yeast in the body, which can lead to the yeast infection known as Candidiasis. Fungal yeast thrives when high glucose foods are eaten and can cause intense sugar cravings. An overgrowth of fungal yeast can also occur when antibiotics or oral contraception are taken regularly, or when undigested food ferments in the intestinal tract. The most significant symptoms of yeast infection include thrush, wind, bloating, mouth ulcers, bad breath, skin problems, plantar wart flare-ups and mood swings.

Refined sugar

Refined sugar, for the purpose of this book, refers to any sugar that has been processed to create a product dramatically different from its original form. It has little or no nutrient content, in some cases contains chemicals from processing and most times has a very high Glycaemic Index (GI). Each glucose-producing food is given a GI, this indicates how quickly food is converted to glucose in the blood – the lower the number the better.

You can still have your cake (or berry tart) and eat it too!

The good news is, that just because you have cut out gluten, yeast, dairy, eggs and refined sugar, it doesn't mean you have to go without beautiful, decadent desserts and sweet treats. Just imagine, gloriously melt-in-your-mouth yummy food actually being good for you!

Our body converts carbohydrates to glucose to give us energy. Our pancreas produces insulin to manage this glucose. Eating too many sugary foods overworks the pancreas as a lot of insulin is required to keep blood sugar levels stable. Diabetes can be the result of eating too many high GI foods which can create high blood sugar levels.

Intolerances to sugar can cause tummy cramps, bloating, wind, nausea, vomiting, thrush, chest and viral infections, attention problems and depression. If symptoms persist after eliminating sucrose (refined sugar) from the diet, this could indicate problems processing other sugars such as fructose found in fruit and vegetables. Some other names for refined sugar listed on processed food packets include: cane sugar, beet sugar, maltose (malt sugar), maltodextrin, high fructose corn syrup and agave nectar.

By eliminating gluten, egg, dairy, yeast and refined sugar from my diet, I felt like I was giving my immune system a break and the inflammation had a chance to ease.

When I started reintroducing foods back into my diet, my body became super sensitive. I found that I reacted quickly to the foods causing me problems, making it clear which foods to either cut out or reduce. Most of my symptoms were alleviated and some went away completely when I stopped eating gluten, yeast, dairy, eggs and refined sugar for three whole months - Halleluiah! This was such a relief and I was so encouraged by my body's response, it inspired me to continue healing myself this way.

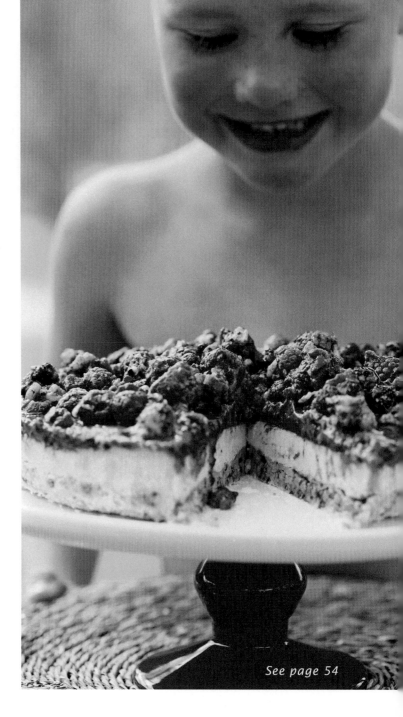

See page 54

There are many methods documented that explain how to reintroduce particular foods back into your diet after you've been on an elimination diet. I tried to keep things simple and doable as I had three small children at the time. I reintroduced one type of eliminated food for a couple of days and observed the symptoms. When I felt satisfied with the result, I took myself back off that food, waited a few days then tried the next food and so on. From these results I built a picture of which foods affected me immediately and which gave me grief for hours and sometimes days after. I discovered there were some foods I could handle in small amounts, provided I didn't overdo them. These foods have become my treat foods even though they aren't always sweet.

global Health

Taking a quick glance at global health, or lack of it, one can see that there are some scary trends emerging in relation to the overall health of our world's population and the prevalence of a handful of diseases that are rapidly growing into epidemics. The biggies are Cancer, Cardiovascular disease, Diabetes and Obesity. I could provide a long list of statistics on each disease, however I'll just give an overview from the World Health Organisation's website, which I think is all we need to get the picture.

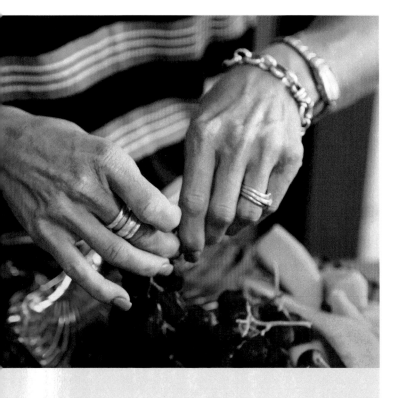

Currently about 7.6 million people globally, die from Cancer each year, with this number predicted to increase to 13.1 million by 2030.

Diabetes-related deaths are due to increase by more than 50% worldwide in the next 10 years.

Cardiovascular disease, which includes all diseases involving the heart and blood vessels, was the cause of 30% of all global deaths in 2008. In 2030 it is predicted that 23 million people will die from Cardiovascular disease.

Obesity is on the increase with 2.8 million people dying on the planet each year as a result of being overweight or obese. It also appears to be the most preventable cause of death.

The good news is, research has shown that the chance of dying from one or more of these diseases is reduced if we regularly exercise, eat vegetables and fruit, don't smoke, drink less alcohol and reduce stress.

Millions and millions of people all around the world are dying or being affected by these diseases. Sadly they seem to be on the increase even though there are millions and millions of dollars raised to research their causes, find cures and provide specialist care for patients. Why is it that developed countries like Australia don't have a more preventative approach to disease? I'd like to see more energy, time and money spent encouraging kids to drink fresh water, eat fresh wholefood and play more outdoor sports so disease and obesity rates may be lowered.

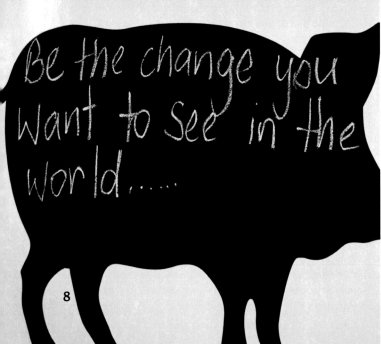

Be the change you want to see in the world......

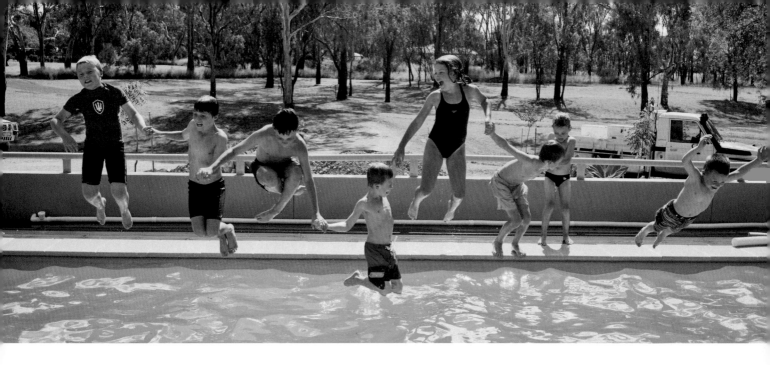

Great work is being carried out by a growing number of proactive groups who are encouraging us to grow and eat fresh food. At the same time though, companies selling processed food sponsor major national sporting events as well as our kids local sport. I believe this is giving our children mixed messages about how to be healthy.

I'd love to see school canteens, sporting organisations, the media and government place greater emphasis on the benefits of eating more fresh wholefood and less processed food. I believe our communities will reap the rewards as our children thrive and achieve great things by eating food their growing bodies need. Who knows, even world peace may be achieved if we all eat well!

It's a sad fact that in some parts of the world children are dying from starvation and in other parts they are dying of overeating. I even read a report that in some developing countries, where the traditional diet is being replaced with a more western diet, it is not uncommon to find one family member malnourished and another obese.

The recurring factors influencing the onset of all the illnesses above are unhealthy diet and lifestyle trends. To reverse these trends, it's clear we really do need to exercise, eat more vegetables and fruit, stop smoking, reduce alcohol consumption and eat less processed, high fat, high sugar foods.

If we stop exercising and nourishing our bodies with healthy food and drink, we seem to become blind to the signs and symptoms in front of us that can lead to disease if neglected.

In my case, I am now convinced that I had some susceptibility to disease before I was born. Throughout my life I think there have been factors that taunted that susceptibility and eventually eroded any defence mechanisms my body may have had to fight disease. These factors joined forces with the negative effects of the foods I was eating, which I now know I am intolerant to. Finally my body couldn't fight the good fight anymore and Scleroderma manifested itself within me.

Scleroderma is an autoimmune disease which causes one's own immune system to attack itself. This damages connective tissue, affecting the skin, joints and sometimes the organs. This damaged tissue hardens, making the skin feel tight and dry and the joints feel sore and swollen.

I knew nothing about autoimmune diseases until I was diagnosed in 2001. I now hear about them all the time. Some of the more common diseases are Lupus, Grave's disease, Hashimoto's disease, Rheumatoid Arthritis, Type 1 Diabetes (requiring insulin injections), Multiple Sclerosis and Sjogren's syndrome. There seem to be more of them popping up each year as well as illnesses now being labelled as autoimmune diseases.

I have not been able to find any documented medical cure for Scleroderma. I do find it interesting though that throughout the years, as I have sought to find key medical information to help me feel better, there have been very few neon flashing references to the fact that diet can have a dramatic impact on the severity of its symptoms.

I now regularly meet people who suffer from autoimmune-related illnesses. Many are yet to experiment with diet to find which foods make them feel great and which exacerbate their symptoms. They are encouraged by the prospect that relief can come from tweaks to their daily menu.

Family & Community

I started cooking when I was on a chair in front of the stove at the age of about nine, concocting meals for the family. I didn't have a clue about ingredients and I used all the herbs and spices in the rack. I remember Uncle Charlie lovingly saying to me once, 'Hey, you don't put cinnamon in spaghetti bolognese'. This didn't seem to worry anyone in my immediate family, especially Mum who eats to live, whereas I live to eat. The point is, Mum allowed me to cook. She allowed the cinnamon in the dish and she turned a blind eye to the mess and the waste when I used to experiment. For this I am very grateful. Although Mum had little passion for cooking, she gave me the opportunity to develop my passion from a very young age.

Guided by insights that my health situation has given me, it is my passion for nutritious food I now hope to foster in my own children. At every stage of this journey I tell our kids why we are doing something and I try to back this up with some evidence. One example is that my second son becomes very congested with mucus and coughs at night if he drinks a glass of cow's milk. So when the coughing starts he knows what I am going to say. He now drinks water or rice milk quite happily and his coughing symptoms have disappeared.

Thankfully our kids are active and I try to explain whenever I can that if they want to achieve well at school and on the sporting field their bodies need healthy high-performance food.

I also tell our kids that good food helps you to feel happy, which helps you think more positively and that leads to a winning attitude.

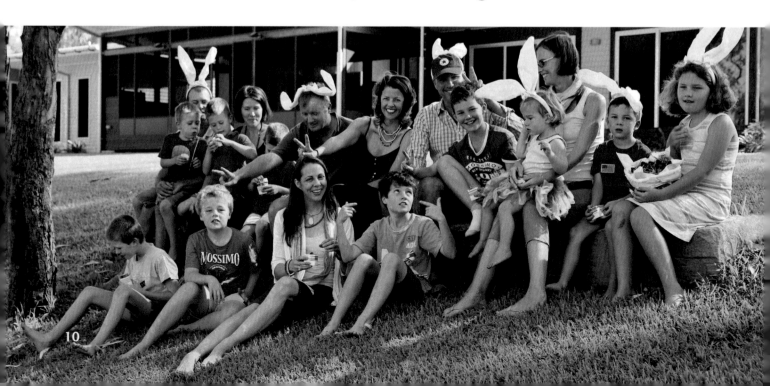

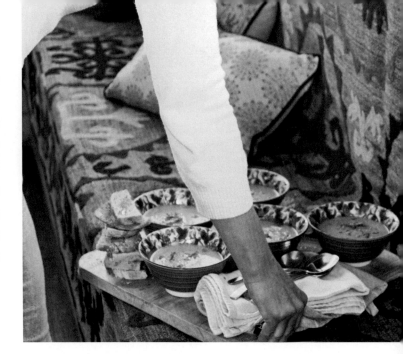

I have always loved everything involved with food, buying ingredients, cooking, eating out, new food innovations, all of it – love it! Chopping, cooking and creating food makes me extremely happy. I'm always inspired when I have time to potter in the kitchen. I also love travelling and when I travel somewhere I can't wait to get to where I'm going, to see what sort of food they eat there.

For the most part our children seem happy with our family's take on food and thankfully most of our friends have a similar take on theirs. However sometimes our kids feel a little self-conscious about the lunch they take to school. I often encourage them to simply enjoy what's in their lunchboxes and I am inspired by how they're learning to handle comments about their food in a positive way.

I have faith that in the future even more families will have a better understanding of the value of nutritious food and will reap the benefits as their children thrive.

From time to time we take our kids to a fast-food restaurant and sometimes they have a pie and a soft drink from the sports canteen (let's hope this isn't always possible at sporting venues). Occasionally they also buy lollies with their pocket money. I cringe when they do this but guided by the many stories and information they have heard from me over the years, they are becoming aware of how they feel after eating some of these foods and they're able to verbalise their symptoms. More often now our kids are making healthier choices when we provide them with these opportunities.

I also find it helps our children take ownership of their health by helping to menu plan, buy groceries, cook meals and prepare their own lunchboxes. I have always let them cut up food, cook whenever possible and grab a shopping basket to buy their own ingredients after finding a recipe they like. What I have loved about our babies sitting at the kitchen bench whilst I prepare meals, is that they get to taste and experiment with food.

They would eat half the raw veggies before they went in the saucepan and our older kids still reach for them as they walk past the kitchen. Try leaving raw, cut-up veggies on the kitchen bench half an hour before you put them in the pot and see how many are left when you go to cook them! You may be surprised.

Meal times are most enjoyable at our house when the whole family sits together. I find it's an ideal time to monitor our children's appetites and teach table manners. It's also a great place to encourage open communication by sharing a joke, a funny story from the day or some important news. Some of my loveliest childhood memories involve a family meal and a festive occasion.

Our food is always made tastier by the warm, loving environment created by the family and friends we share our meals with.

Vegetable and herb gardens are another great way to nurture the family's love of fresh wholefood by getting the kids to help plant, tend and pick their own produce. It is also a lovely way to teach children how much energy and effort goes into growing food. Our kids are always happy to pick something from the garden to go in our dinner and they seem a little excited to know they have contributed to the family meal in some way.

Habits we encourage during our family meal:

- Thank the farmer, the gardener and the cook.
- Avoid drinking cold drinks with hot meals.
- Chew food well to assist with digestion.
- Turn the TV off and focus on each other.

my HealinG Journey

Reflection and research has enabled me to draw some preliminary conclusions as to why I may have Scleroderma. I now think the cause involved a combination of the chemical load I had collected and carried throughout my life, personality traits that made me stress, the types of foods I had eaten prior to diagnosis and of course, alcohol.

Firstly, let me put you in the picture as to why I think chemicals have played a part in my illness. Throughout the last 13 years I have consulted on and off with alternative health practitioners and most have said that I have chemicals in my system handed to me by my farming ancestors.

Whilst I am sure I am not the first country baby to be born with an inherited chemical load, the following facts may have started the chemicals compounding a little quicker than normal.

I was born because of my parent's heartfelt desire to have another baby. Having experienced many miscarriages, in order to stay pregnant with me, my mother was regularly injected with drugs so her body would not reject me in utero. Luckily the drugs worked and I was born but it may be that this, together with my inherited chemicals, compromised my immune system from birth.

I grew up on the banks of the Boomi River, in between Boomi and Mungindi, on a sheep and wheat property. Later as a young teen my family moved to the mountains near Allora, Queensland where my father grew mostly summer crops and fattened cattle on the beautiful slopes near the Goomburra Valley. I am a descendant of seven

generations of farming stock. Agriculture is in my blood and quite literally in my genes. With the help of my mother and father, I have researched the types of chemicals we have used over the years in our agricultural practices and found worrying information.

Of the globally recognised Persistent Organic Pollutants (POPs), also known as the 'Dirty Dozen', I have been directly exposed to at least half of them, including sheep dips containing arsenic. At the moment there may be no official proven links between exposure to these chemicals and the incidence of Scleroderma, however one can't say this sort of exposure is a good thing. Through my research I have discovered there's a strong possibility that the exposure to some of these chemicals is linked to the very symptoms I now suffer from.

On reflection, another factor that may have contributed to me initially developing Scleroderma symptoms was the way I handled emotional stress.

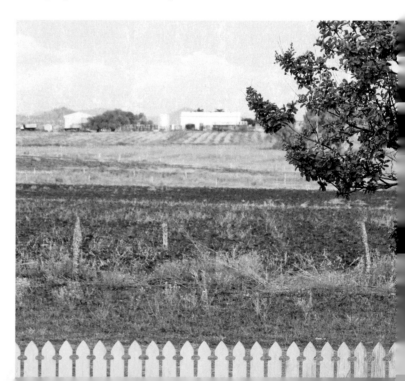

I am learning as I get older, that sometimes when we want to know the answers to some of those perplexing questions about our life, questions like 'why me?' and 'how did I get to this point?', we have to reflect on our past. This reflection has given me insight into some of the people, experiences and events that have shaped the person I am today. Some good, some challenging!

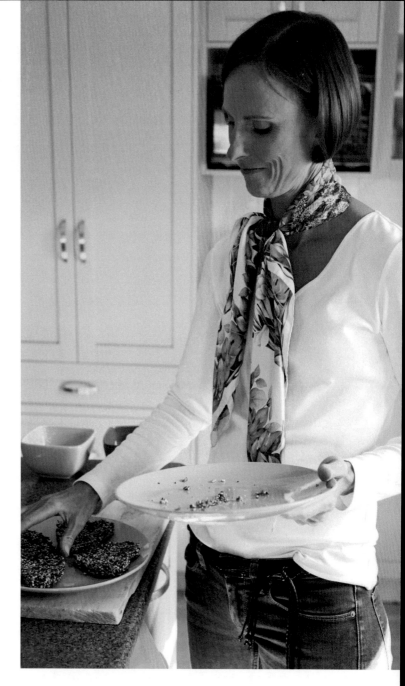

From the age of 12, after I went to boarding school and left my idyllic, safe country childhood behind, I started to suffer from extremely low self-esteem which caused me a lot of anxiety. In year 9 and 10 I started smoking and drinking alcohol to help me feel strong, happy and confident. By year 12 I was struggling. I was bullied by a small group of girls in my year and I didn't have the courage or the conviction to stand up for myself. This made me feel even more insecure.

When I experienced bouts of self-doubt and anxiety, I didn't react by kicking something or by screaming and yelling. Instead, I swallowed down these negative thoughts and feelings and I created ways to hide them by acting tough and behaving rebelliously.

Throughout early adulthood my dependence on alcohol and cigarettes grew. An after-effect of drinking heavily meant I ate badly. Every day I would eat some sort of junk food and if a hangover was really bad I would drink more alcohol.

It wasn't long after I met my husband, the love of my life, that my health started to decline rapidly. Perhaps it's no coincidence that at the time he was a cotton agronomist and would come home each night smelling of chemicals. I was also not in a good frame of mind. I wasn't enjoying my job and I was negative about many other aspects of my life. One morning after a particularly heavy binge-drinking weekend I woke doubled over in pain. An ultrasound revealed chronic constipation. Weeks later I developed puffy, tight and painful hands and feet. Our GP referred me to a Rheumatologist who diagnosed me.

After my diagnosis, I wandered through life for about a year feeling sorry for myself. These feelings were not good for my symptoms and I soon realised that I felt sicker when I thought about what I had. My specialist told us to start trying for a family as there could be difficulties falling pregnant and miscarriage was common in Scleroderma patients. Luckily this wasn't the case for us.

After we had our first and second babies, I realised how important it was for me to be as healthy as possible in order to care for my family. It was also important to me to delay taking drugs to alleviate my symptoms so I started visiting alternative health practitioners. I eventually found one who motivated me to heal myself naturally.

It was this healer's advice to take myself off gluten, yeast, dairy, eggs, refined sugar and of course, alcohol for three months, that has changed my life forever.

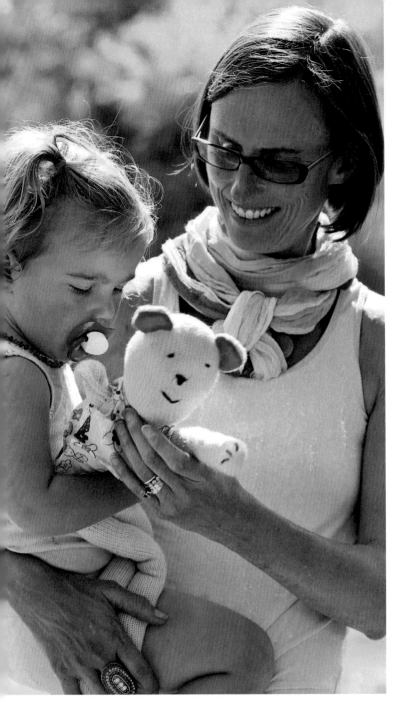

I now have an abundance of energy and I love my roles as wife and mum. I know I wouldn't be where I am today if I still ate and drank the way I used to.

I now see my Scleroderma has forced me to make better life choices and I would like my children to benefit from my lessons so that inappropriate food won't contribute to any genetic predisposition they may have to autoimmunity. My minimised Scleroderma symptoms now simmer in the background as a constant reminder to me that I must nurture and respect my body so I can be the best Felicity Philp in the world.

Before I changed my diet:

I had puffy hands and feet, aching arthritic joints, heartburn, cramping and restless legs, headaches, subcutaneous calcinosis (calcium deposits under the skin near bones and joints), dry eyes, dry mouth and nasal passages, frequent bouts of Candidiasis, extreme tiredness, no libido, bouts of depression, poor self-esteem, sugar and wheat cravings, premenstrual tension (PMT) and severe abdominal pain, constipation alternating with diarrhoea, bloating, wind and inflamed psoriasis.

After I changed my diet:

I now find I have fresher breath and no foot or underarm odour, PMT and abdominal pain are very moderate, I have drastically reduced soreness and stiffness in the joints, cramping and restless legs have disappeared, bloating and wind has eased and bowel movements are more consistent. I experience no Candidiasis, my subcutaneous calcinosis has all but disappeared, my skin is clearer, hair and nails stronger, eyes brighter, psoriasis has improved, I have no food cravings and my mental clarity is excellent.

After three months on this elimination diet and after the reintroduction of each food type, there was evidence that I couldn't tolerate some foods. I now know I can't eat gluten, yeast and refined sugar and I can tolerate only small amounts of egg and dairy. Today I still experience symptoms of my condition, but for most of them a great edge has been taken off their severity. In comparison to how I felt before I changed my diet, I now feel fantastic. A significant change has been my ability to identify and deal with other stress triggers that lead to health setbacks. I now avoid these situations as much as possible. I find my head makes good choices when my body is feeling great. With a better diet and a positive outlook on myself and my life, I feel like I can do anything I set my mind to.

In a nutshell, by improving the food I ate, I had removed the many negative reactions going on inside my body. This freed up my mind and gave me back the energy I needed to think about more positive, creative ways to live my life.

Plan & Prep

The first step I took that really kickstarted my healing journey was to reorganise my kitchen. This made it easier to stick to the new elimination diet. I set a start date, went through the pantry and hid or boxed up any ingredients that didn't fit the criteria. I set about stocking my pantry with appropriate ingredients that I put into sections for baking, quick snacks and meals. This still helps me when I am really hungry and need a quick healthy snack or meal to get on with my day.

The ingredients that can take up a lot of room in the fridge are the condiments. Also if you look at the ingredients panels on these products you'll notice a lot of nasties and really - if it can live in your fridge for two years, it's not food. I ditched these items and most of the food I eat now is perishable, e.g. vegetables and fruit, so I allow plenty of space in the fridge for these foods. By the time I need to do a grocery shop, the fridge is pretty bare.

As a result of the reorganisation of my kitchen, I now keep wholefood snacks like fresh and dried fruit, nuts, seeds and crackers visible and accessible so the family can munch on them easily throughout the day. I also keep homemade healthier treat foods like biscuits and cakes in a less accessible position in the pantry so they aren't eaten as regularly as the wholefood snacks.

I've found it's important to be organised, menu plan and shop accordingly. It's when I am having a super busy day and I'm not organised with snacks, that the temptation creeps in to have something not in the plan. I now take a packed lunchbox with me when out and about as it can be hard to find just the right kind of meal from café menus when you're trying to avoid certain ingredients.

Equipment Required:

I like to keep things simple and affordable so most of my cooking involves a bowl and spoon. If you have the following items in your kitchen then you can make everything in this book with ease.

- An oven and cooktop. All baked recipes in this book are cooked on a fan-forced setting.
- A food processor. I use a small one as it chops small quantities well and I do two batches of processing for larger quantities.

- A handheld electric stick mixer.
- A set of scales. I prefer the exactness of digital.
- A set of quality measuring cups (in Australia 1 cup is 250 ml). Be mindful that some countries measure cups differently. Avoid using cheap inaccurate plastic measuring cups.
- A set of quality measuring spoons (in Australia 1 tablespoon is 20 ml and 1 teaspoon is 5 ml). Be mindful that some countries measure spoons differently as well.
- Wooden or stainless steel spoons, if possible.
- A good selection of stainless steel bowls.
- A set of good quality, non-coated saucepans and a casserole dish with a lid.
- A good quality, non-coated frying pan.
- A selection of baking trays, loaf tins and round spring-form tins.
- Baking paper. I use unbleached chlorine-free.

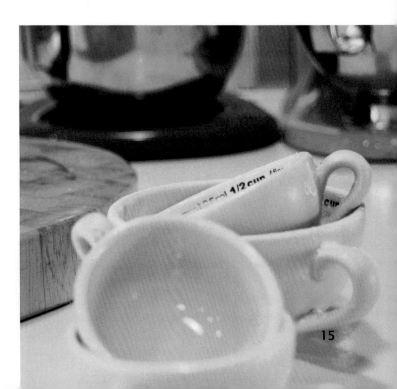

InGreDients

I feel great when my pantry is fully stocked with all my favourite healthy foods. I have found we eat less when I use nutritious, good quality ingredients. This makes it possible to feed our family of six a healthy balanced diet while relying on one income. Over the last five years I've learnt so much about food - good and bad. If I found some ingredients were over-processed or contained unsuitable additives, I sourced a better alternative. The list below includes the best pantry ingredients I have found to date.

Activated nuts & seeds

'Activating' is the process of making the nutrients in nuts and seeds more readily available to the body. The process involves soaking the nuts or seeds in water (or salt water), then draining and dehydrating them at a low temperature. Basically the process of germination begins at this stage, breaking down the phytic acid and enzyme inhibitors, both of which require the body to work very hard to digest the nuts or seeds. I also love the crunch factor of activated nuts and seeds.

Almond milk

Almond milk is made from ground almonds and water. It is more nutritious than rice milk and contains no lactose. It does however contain protein and omega 3 fatty acids. Choose an almond milk that has the least additives. Makes great custard.

Apple cider vinegar

Apple cider vinegar is made from the fermented juice of apples and has many reported health benefits. Try to find organic, unfiltered vinegar containing the 'mother', as it has more minerals, vitamins and enzymes than most commercial brands. I use it with extra-virgin olive oil for a quick salad dressing most days.

Arrowroot

Arrowroot is the starch from the rootstock of several tropical plants. It is useful to thicken sauces, especially those containing acidic food as well as delicately flavoured sauces. Arrowroot can tolerate long cooking times and freezing. It also helps to stop ice crystals forming in ice creams. Arrowroot is sometimes mislabelled as tapioca flour and vice versa.

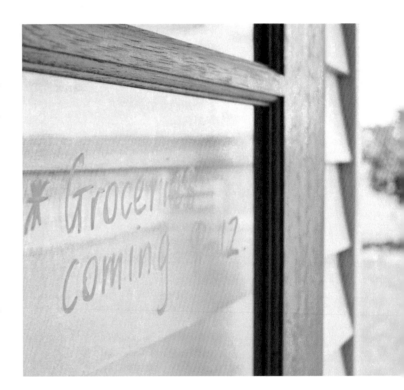

Baking powder & Sodium bicarbonate

Both are used as raising agents. Sodium bicarbonate (bicarb soda) requires an acid such as apple cider vinegar to help baked goods rise. Choose brands free of aluminium, chlorine and gluten.

Besan flour

This gluten-free flour is also known as chickpea or garbanzo flour. It is made from ground, dried or roasted chickpeas and is high in carbohydrates and protein. It binds well and fortunately loses some of its bitterness during cooking. Mix with water to make unleavened pancakes (crêpe-style).

Braggs All Purpose Seasoning

Braggs All Purpose Seasoning is made from soybeans and water. It is great to add depth of flavour to many savoury dishes without the use of additive-laden sauces and stock powders. In addition to this wonderful seasoning, Braggs have a wide range of healthy nutritious foods which includes their Organic Sprinkle.

Buckwheat flour

Buckwheat flour (not related to wheat) has a nutty, earthy flavour. It is packed full of goodness as it is rich in fibre, protein, calcium, phosphorus, zinc and the list goes on. This flour is better in baked goods when mixed together with nut meals and other flours like quinoa and besan. Buckwheat flour also makes lovely pancakes when a little arrowroot flour is added to the pancake mix.

Cacao powder

Cacao powder (raw) is one of the by-products of pulverising the cacao bean, the other by-product being cacao butter. Cacao powder is rich in flavour and due to low temperature processing, retains it's vitamins, minerals and powerful antioxidants. Good quality cacao powder is free of chemicals and a great source of protein, B vitamins, calcium, chromium, zinc, iron and more. Cacao also contains magnesium which assists in relaxing muscles and reducing stress. Look for cacao products made from the superior criollo variety of cacao bean.

Cacao nibs & wafers

Cacao nibs are shelled and crushed cacao beans. They are nutritious and high in antioxidants. For extra-special occasions I buy pure cacao wafers which come in little bite-sized buttons. They contain the cacao butter and the cacao powder before they are separated. They are great for making quick additive-free chocolate treats.

Chia seeds

This wonderful superfood, originating from Central America, has the highest known plant source of omega 3. These seeds contain powerful antioxidants, vitamin A, vitamin B12, vitamin C, potassium, phosphorus, folate, zinc, iron and calcium. They are also a great source of protein and fibre. Add to drinks, breakfast dishes, puddings and breads. One teaspoon is the recommended daily dose for maximum health benefits.

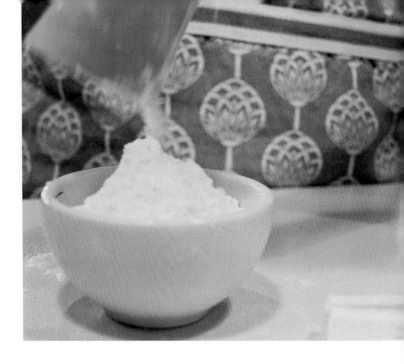

Coconut oil

Coconut oil, also known as coconut butter, is a healthy saturated oil, converted into energy by the liver rather than being stored as fat. Countless benefits include weight loss, managing Type 2 Diabetes, stopping sugar cravings and boosting the immune system with its antifungal, antiviral and antibacterial properties. Coconut oil cooks at high temperatures, unlike other oils which are reported to oxidise and create free radicals at high temperatures.

Coconut sugar

This crystallised nectar from the coconut palm tree blossom is a beautiful toffee-flavoured natural sweetener. It has a low GI of 35 and is very nutritious as it contains protein, potassium, magnesium, phosphorus, zinc and iron. Use the same quantity as you would for refined sugar.

Cornflour

Cornflour (or corn starch) thickens sauces, gravies and custards. It breaks down and thins when cooked for long periods or when mixed with acidic ingredients. Upon thawing food containing cornflour, the food can become sticky and moist. Ensure the cornflour you choose is gluten-free.

Extra-virgin olive oil

Cold pressed extra-virgin olive oil is the oil from the first pressing of the olives and contains the most nutrients. It is high in oleic acid which is believed to protect the heart and reduce the risk of cancer. Buy in small quantities and store in a cool, dark place. Use fresh and never heat beyond its smoke point.

Flaxseeds

Flaxseeds (also known as linseeds) have antioxidant qualities and are high in fibre, protein, calcium and a plethora of other micronutrients. Some reports state that eating flaxseeds reduces the severity of Diabetes by stabilising blood sugar levels. I love the nuttiness of these seeds and use them in breads, cakes and snacks.

Gluten-free custard powder

Gluten-free custard powder is available in a few different brands. I always reduce the liquid amount they suggest by a few tablespoons so the custard is richer and thicker.

Gluten-free flours

When I first started out on the gluten-free track I used premixed gluten-free self-raising flours. I don't use many of these flours now because they contain the additive 466, which is a thickening agent listed by naturalhealthclinic.com.au as an additive for children to avoid. For the recipes in this book I have used Orgran gluten-free self-raising flour as it is 466 free. After some experimentation, I have now discovered the flavour of baked goods can be improved by mixing flours with certain characteristics. Two handy premixed plain flour products from Bob's Red Mill are 'Garbanzo and Fava Flour' and 'All Purpose Baking Flour'.

Gluten-free oats

Also known as uncontaminated oats. It appears that some people with Coeliac disease can eat uncontaminated oat products. Oats in their pure form are in fact gluten-free. Mass-produced oat products are contaminated during harvest, transport and processing. Look for uncontaminated gluten-free oats in your local health food shop. When eating oats make sure you have plenty of fluids with them. When I first gave up gluten, I did not know about oats in their pure form and did not eat them. I now enjoy a good bowl of porridge a couple of times a week.

Honey

Honey is produced by bees using the nectar of plants. It has a similar sweetness to refined sugar with some antioxidant properties. Its GI ranges from 31 to 78 depending on the variety. Blended honeys have a higher GI. I use yellow box honey which has a GI of about 35. Look for raw organic honey as there is minimal heat used to extract this honey from the comb. It is this heat that devalues the nutrients in the finished product.

Lucuma powder

An exotic dried and ground Peruvian fruit, high in nutrients and great to enhance desserts.

Macadamia oil

A beautiful, nutty oil from the Australian macadamia nut. Like extra-virgin olive oil, it is high in oleic acid. It has a high smoke point and is great in biscuits, cakes and salads. Macadamia oil is also reported to have anti-inflammatory properties.

Maple syrup

Maple syrup is the sap from the maple tree and is twice as sweet as refined sugar. It is reduced by heat until it is thick and syrupy. This syrup contains significant amounts of potassium and calcium, with smaller amounts of manganese and zinc. It has a GI of 54 and some antioxidant qualities. Choose 100% pure maple syrup.

Nut butters

100% nuts ground into a paste. Available in different nut varieties.

Nuttelex

Nuttelex is the best butter replacement I've found so far for the recipes in this book. The manufacturer states it is vegan and virtually trans-fat free.

Polenta

Coarsley-ground yellow or white cornmeal cooked with water and/or stock and herbs. This is a great winter comfort food to have with casseroles.

Pomegranate molasses

A Middle Eastern syrup made from reduced pomegranate juice. Great as an alcohol replacement in cakes and drinks.

Quinoa

Quinoa is a very nutritious gluten-free grain with more protein than any other grain. High in fibre, iron, B vitamins, calcium, magnesium and vitamin E, it also has a low GI. I use it to replace cracked wheat and cous cous.

Rice crumbs

Rice crumbs are made from baked rice. Source brown rice crumbs rather than white as the latter are more processed. Rice crumbs are a great replacement for bread crumbs containing gluten.

Rice milk

Rice milk is produced using mainly brown rice. It contains some calcium and no lactose which can cause tummy upsets. Rice milk has a sweet taste and is a good cow's milk replacement most of the time. Choose a brand with the least additives.

Salt

Choose a natural sea or rock salt free from anti-caking agents containing gluten. Common table salt is heated to such high temperatures during processing, the molecular structure of the sodium chloride is altered making it harder for the body to process. Common table salt also contains chemicals and is linked to the acceleration of many modern ailments including heart disease. It is added to many processed foods and is excessively high in take-away foods. My everyday salt is the gorgeous pink fine Himalayan rock salt as it contains the most trace elements and minerals of all the salts. Its mineral composition exactly replicates that of the fluids in our body, which adds weight to the theory that our bodies do need natural salt.

Soy milk & tofu

I try to steer clear of soy products. I have read about modern processing and how shortcuts in production could be creating inferior soy products that may be a threat to our health. However, I trialled different milks for the mayonnaise recipe and good quality, gluten-free soy milk worked the best. Tofu is an ancient Asian food made from coagulated soy milk pressed into blocks. It is high in protein, iron and sometimes calcium, depending on how it is processed. Tofu is available firm or silken.

Stevia

Stevia is a natural sweetener made from the stevia plant. It can be up to 300 times sweeter than refined sugar. I personally don't enjoy the stevia flavour in food but I love the liquid drops in my soda water with a twist of lime.

Sulphite-free dried fruit

Sulphites (220-228) are additives used to preserve food and they are extremely high in some dried fruit, especially apricots. The recommended daily intake for an average 10 year old is 15 mg of sulphites or one dried apricot. Choose dried fruit products labelled organic as they should be sulphite-free. Sulphites are connected with asthma attacks and are found in many foods and drinks e.g. children's snack foods, health and breakfast bars, cured meats, alcoholic ciders and wines.

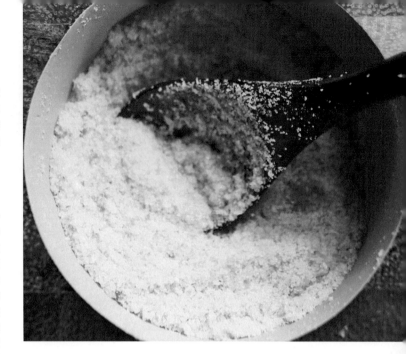

Tahini

Tahini is a paste made from ground sesame seeds. It binds ingredients and adds depth of flavour to dips and sweets. It is a great source of calcium, protein, copper, manganese and omega 3 and 6 fatty acids. Choose unhulled, raw tahini as the fibre provides added health benefits.

Tamari

Tamari is made from fermented soybeans. It is dark and rich without the overpowering nature of standard soy sauce, which can contain gluten, refined sugar, alcohol and additives. Check the label because not all tamari is wheat-free.

Tapioca flour

Tapioca flour is made from the root starches found in the cassava plant. It is a good binder and is also great to give cakes and breads a bit of springiness, or to give pizza a crispy crust. Tapioca flour doesn't handle long cooking times, freezing or acidic conditions well.

Tinned foods

When buying tinned food, look for tins free of the carbon-based synthetic compound BPA.

Xanthan gum

Xanthan gum is made from fermented corn and is used a lot in gluten-free cooking to help thicken and bind. It prevents baked goods from crumbling. If you discover you have problems with corn products then you can substitute (for equal quantities) guar gum, which is made from a bean-like legume.

Breakfast

When I used to eat cereal and milk brekkys, I found myself ravenous by 10 am and hankering for a processed carbohydrate fix. I feel great when I start my day with a bowl of fresh fruit followed by one of the breakfast recipes in this section and I never have hunger pains before lunch time now. I vary this second course so I don't get tired of the same thing. The Bircher-Style Muesli is my fave, while our kids love the Potato Hashies and would eat them every morning if they could.

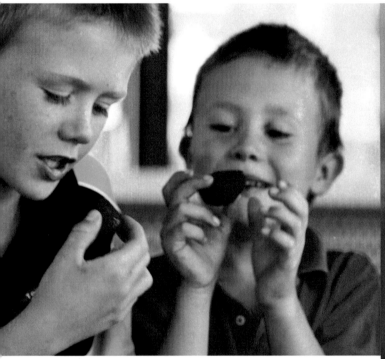

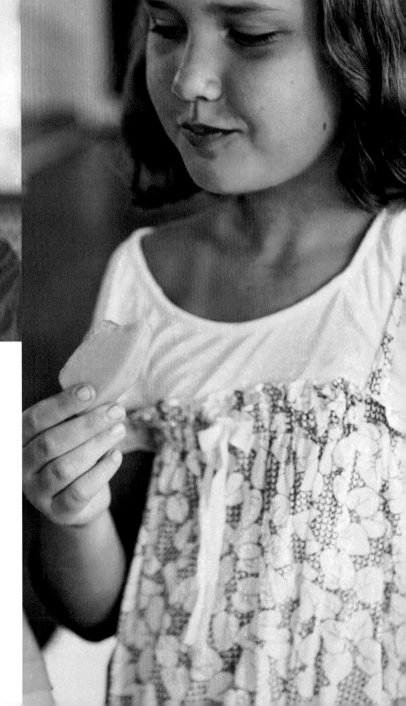

fruit platter

At our house every morning I cut up a large platter of mixed seasonal fruit for the family. Interestingly, at this time of the day I enjoy eating my fruit cut up and I understand why my children enjoy this ritual as well. It feels more like a special fruit meal rather than just grabbing an apple and munching on it. The whole platter is eaten every morning so I'm happy that if our kids don't eat another piece of fruit for the rest of the day then at least they have started their day with a great energy hit. While everyone crunches through their fruit I prepare their second course. After this kind of breakfast all our kids happily start their day feeling satisfied, energised and alert.

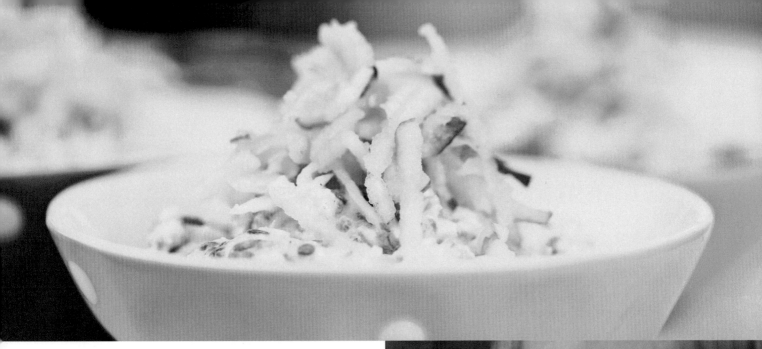

bircher-style muesli

⅓ cup gluten-free rolled oats
⅔ cup almond milk or rice milk
1 tbsp raisins
2 tsp flaxseeds
2 tsp chia seeds
Pinch of mixed spice
Pinch of fine Himalayan rock salt
1 tbsp apple, grated or finely chopped

Place all ingredients except the apple in a small bowl. Cover and refrigerate overnight. Add the apple just before eating. Serves 1.

Great for a quick 'get up and go' brekky.

plum porridge

1 cup gluten-free rolled oats
1 cup rice milk
½ cup water
2 dried pitted prunes
LSA (ground linseeds, sunflower seeds
  and almonds)

Add all ingredients to a saucepan and simmer until thick. Add more rice milk for a thinner porridge. Sprinkle with LSA. Serves 1.

A real comfort breakfast. This meal has satisfied many pregnancy and breastfeeding hunger pains over the years.

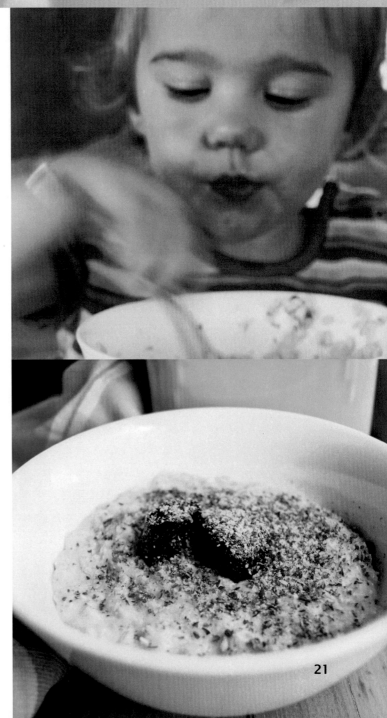

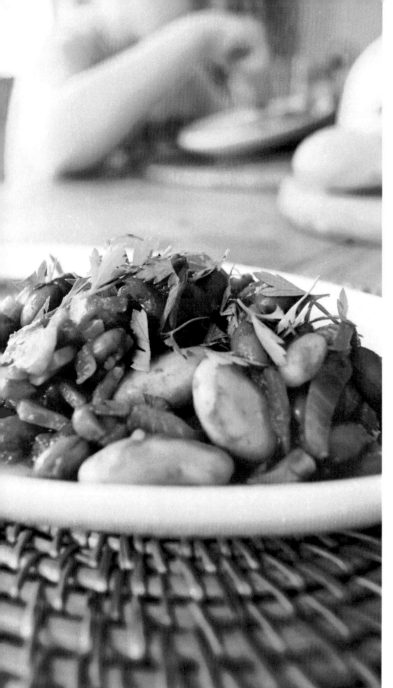

flick's baked beans

2 x 400 g tins borlotti beans (or cannellini
  or butter beans) drained and liquid reserved
400 g tin chopped tomatoes
1 tbsp additive-free tomato paste
1 tbsp honey
4 rashers of bacon, diced (optional)
  (nitrate-free, salted only bacon if possible)
1 medium onion, diced
¼ tsp dried chilli (or to taste)
1 tsp fresh lemon juice
Fine Himalayan rock salt to taste
Cracked black pepper

Fry the bacon and onion in a heavy-based
saucepan over a medium heat until lightly browned
and the onion is soft. Add all other ingredients
and simmer for about 10 minutes. Add some of
the reserved bean juice if it seems dry. Serves 5.

*I have always loved baked beans. They are such a
good, quick, wholesome meal and our family enjoy
eating them any time of the day with a variety of
accompaniments. We are also lucky to have access
to free-range organic pork products and nitrate-
free, salted only bacon. This is well worth tracking
down as it gives the baked beans richness and
depth of flavour.*

*I particularly like my beans served on top of a
baked sweet potato with freshly cracked pepper.
Also great served with toasted Nutty Cornbread
(see page 41).*

tomato zucchini salsa

1 tomato, chopped
1 medium zucchini, grated
2 garlic cloves, crushed
2 tbsp extra-virgin olive oil
¼ cup water
½ tsp ground coriander seeds
Fine Himalayan rock salt to taste
Cracked black pepper

Combine all ingredients in a saucepan and cook
over a medium heat, stirring until the vegetables
are soft and the liquid has reduced. Serve with
Potato Hashies (see page 23).

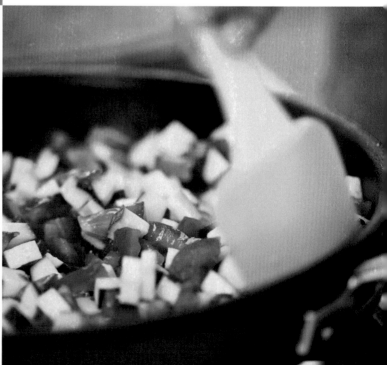

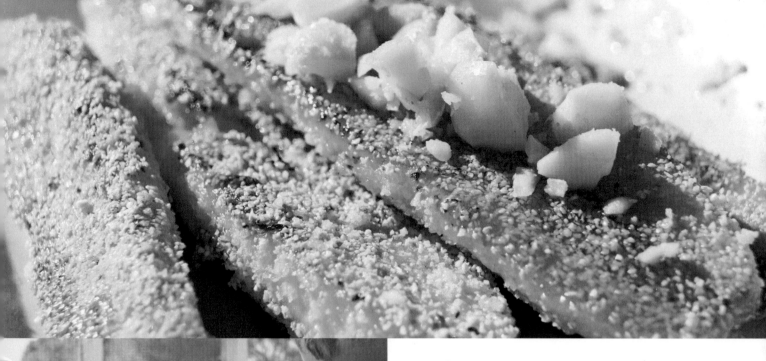

polenta coated bananas

2 ripe bananas
½ cup dry fine polenta
2 tbsp coconut oil
50 g macadamia nuts, roughly chopped
Maple syrup for serving

Heat the oil in a frying pan. Slice the bananas lengthways in half. Coat the bananas in polenta and shallow fry until golden. Remove and drizzle with maple syrup and chopped macadamias. Serves 2.

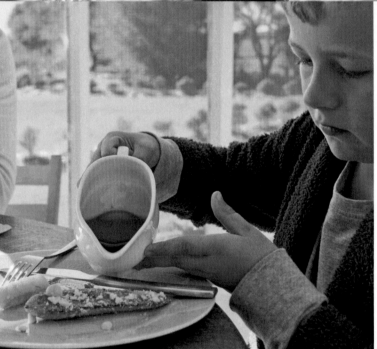

potato hashies

2 medium potatoes, peeled and grated
Extra-virgin olive oil for frying
Fine Himalayan rock salt to taste

Drizzle some oil and salt in the base of a frying pan over a medium heat. Cook 4 pancake-sized portions of the grated potato. Flatten hashies down and tidy the edges to make a round shape. Cook on the first side until golden brown so the hashie can be flipped without falling apart. Cook the other side the same way. Serve with chopped apple and ground cinnamon or Tomato Zucchini Salsa (see page 22). Makes 4 hashies.

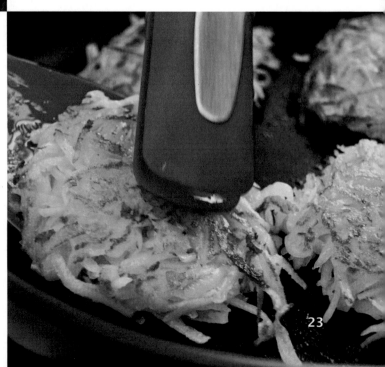

Soups

Soups can be anything you want them to be. I am a bit of a 'throw it all in the pot' type soup maker. I especially love doing this when the grocery items in the fridge start dwindling and I want to use up the remaining vegetables and cold meats. I also like to keep a meat bone of some description on hand so it can go in the pot and add its marrowy goodness to the finished dish. I do love a good recipe as well and the three soups below are my favourites.

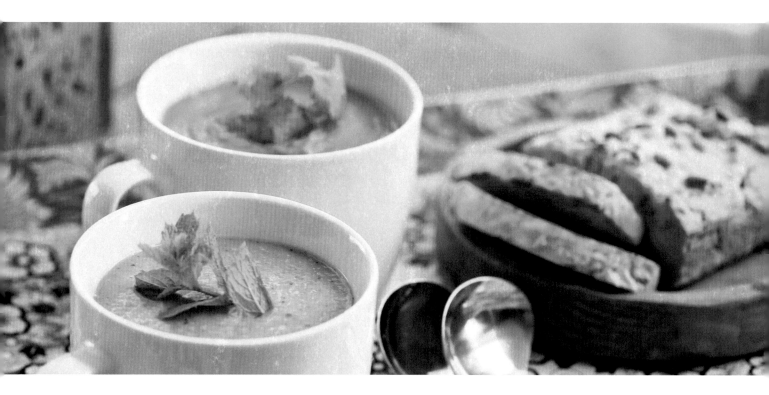

zesty carrot soup

200 g onion, peeled and finely diced
1 tbsp coconut oil
6 large carrots, peeled and finely diced
½ tsp dried chilli flakes (or to taste)
2 cups water
All left over onion and juices from Miranda Kerr's
  Slow Roasted Chicken recipe (see page 34)

In a large heavy-based saucepan over a medium heat, cook the onion in the oil until soft. Add all other ingredients and simmer until the carrot is soft. Purée all ingredients with a stick mixer until smooth. Season to taste. Soup can be served garnished with fresh coriander. Serves 4.

minty pea soup

300 g onion, peeled and finely diced
2 tbsp extra-virgin olive oil
1 medium potato, peeled and cubed
⅓ cup liquid stock (see page 25)
500 g frozen peas
2 tbsp fresh mint, finely chopped

In a large heavy-based saucepan over a medium heat, cook the onion in the oil until soft. Add water, stock and potatoes. Simmer covered until potato is soft. Add the frozen peas and continue to simmer for 5 minutes, then add mint and purée with a stick mixer until smooth. Season to taste. Serves 4.

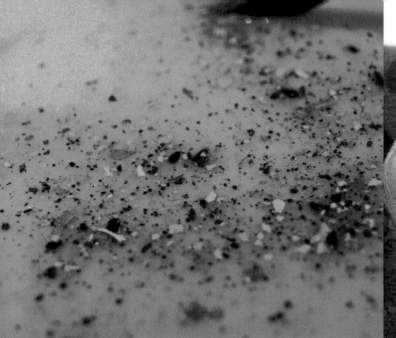

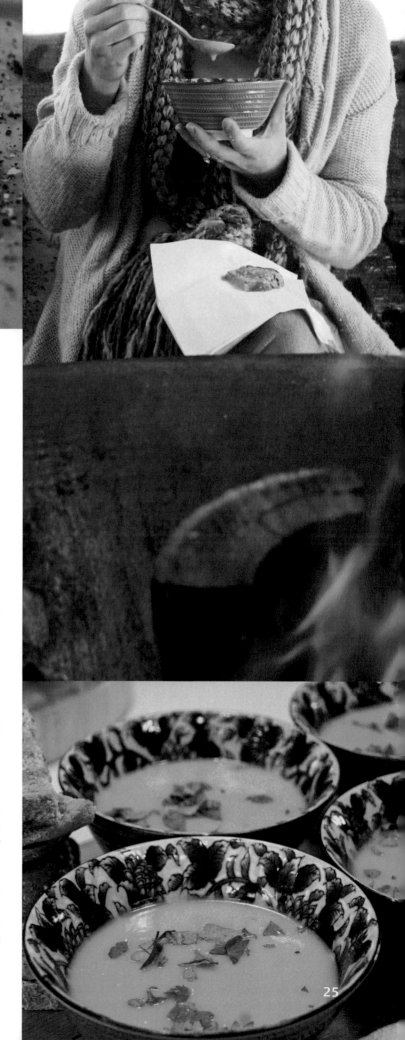

thai-style pumpkin soup

150 g onion, peeled and finely chopped
1 tbsp coconut oil
1.5 kg Kent pumpkin, peeled and chopped
4 cups chicken or vegetable stock
3 garlic cloves
1 heaped tbsp fresh ginger, grated
400 ml tin coconut cream
Fine Himalayan rock salt and chilli flakes to taste
Lime wedges and fresh coriander to garnish

In a large heavy-based saucepan, sauté the onion and garlic in the oil until translucent and sweet. Add the pumpkin and stock then simmer gently until pumpkin is soft. Take off the heat and add the coconut cream and remaining ingredients. Purée with a stick mixer until smooth. Garnish and serve with a lime wedge and fresh coriander. Serves 8 as a main course.

This nourishing winter soup is delicious with toasted gluten-free bread (see page 41).

I love the flavour and texture of Kent pumpkins (also known as Jap) although any kind of pumpkin can be used. Look for pumpkins with buttery yellow spots as these are ripe.

For the stock used in this recipe, you can make your own by boiling chicken bones and vegetables. When I don't have this stock on hand, I use a mix of water, salt, herbs and Braggs All Purpose Seasoning to taste.

SalaDs & LiGht meals

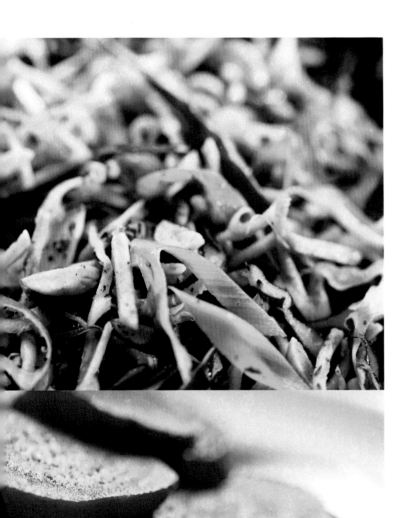

cabbage noodle salad

5-6 cups cabbage, finely shredded
6 spring onions, finely chopped
100 g pine nuts or slivered almonds,
    lightly roasted
1 packet of Chang's gluten-free fried
    rice noodles

DRESSING
¼ cup apple cider vinegar
¼ cup honey
3 tbsp tamari
2 tsp sesame oil
¼ cup extra-virgin olive oil

Combine dressing ingredients in a saucepan
and heat gently until all the ingredients have
amalgamated. Cool and pour over the rest of the
ingredients just before serving, then toss well.

spiced beetroot

400 g beetroot, peeled and sliced
2 cups water
¼ cup apple cider vinegar
1 tsp fine Himalayan rock salt
1 tbsp honey
½ tsp ground cinnamon
½ tsp coriander seeds
½ tsp cardamom seeds
½ tsp caraway seeds
6 whole cloves

Bring all ingredients to the boil in a saucepan with
the lid on. Turn the heat down and simmer with the
lid off for about 15 minutes or until beetroot is soft
and liquid has reduced. Serve when cool.

Having key ingredients on hand to make a good, quick, light meal is important so I don't reach for an unhealthy quick-fix meal. I generally keep cold meat, baked pumpkin, cooked brown rice and quinoa in the fridge for this reason. I love a good salad with lots of interesting bits and bobs including sweet, crisp leaves and some crunchy nuts or seeds, highlighted by simple, flavoursome dressings.

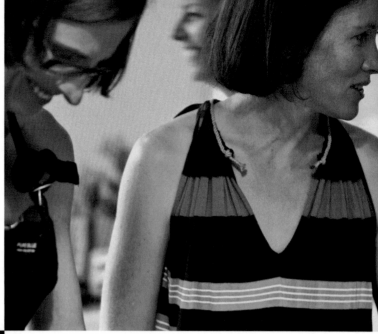

chicken & veg stir-fry

1 kg chicken thigh meat, cut into large chunks with excess fat trimmed
2 tsp fresh ginger, grated
3 garlic cloves, crushed
¼ cup apple cider vinegar
1 tsp fine Himalayan rock salt
1 tbsp coconut oil
1 tsp sesame oil
1 kg mixed vegetables, finely chopped (carrots, capsicum, broccoli, cauliflower, green beans)
100 g bean sprouts
100 g spring onion, finely sliced
2 tsp tamari
4 tbsp honey
1 tsp chilli flakes (optional)
1 cup water
2 tsp arrowroot mixed with a little water

Marinate the chicken in the apple cider vinegar, ginger, garlic and salt for about 2 hours. In a wok, heat the oils on high and cook the chicken in batches until three quarters cooked. Cover and keep warm. Stir-fry the carrots, broccoli and cauliflower in the wok, adding a little more coconut oil if necessary. Then add the capsicum and beans and stir to combine.

When the vegetables are very hot, add the tamari, chilli, honey, water and arrowroot/water mix, then stir thoroughly until the juices thicken. Add the chicken back into the wok and toss through with the vegetables for a couple of minutes. Before serving, add the sprouts and spring onion then give a final toss. Serve on a bed of brown rice. Makes 4-6 portions.

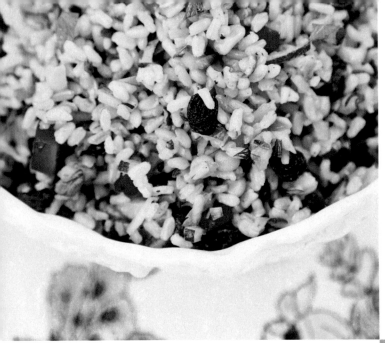

easy rice salad

3 cups brown rice, cooked
½ cup red onion, finely diced
1 green apple, grated
½ cup each of corn kernels, red capsicum, raisins
⅓ cup walnuts, crumbled
2 tbsp fresh parsley, chopped
1 tbsp extra-virgin olive oil
1 garlic clove, crushed in the 1 tbsp of oil
1 tbsp sesame seeds
1 tsp fine Himalayan rock salt
Cracked black pepper

Combine all ingredients and toss well.

baby spinach & pumpkin salad

4 cups baby spinach leaves
2 cups Kent pumpkin pieces, cubed (walnut size)
Extra-virgin olive oil for roasting pumpkin
2 ripe tomatoes, cut into about 8 segments
1 cup cucumber, diced
1 small red onion, finely diced
1 avocado, peeled and cubed
8-10 olives
½ cup pine nuts
½ tsp fine Himalayan rock salt
Cracked black pepper
¾ cup alfalfa sprouts (optional garnish)

Place the cubed pumpkin in a bowl and drizzle with just enough oil to coat the pieces. Sprinkle with salt and toss well. Then pour into a baking dish and level out. Bake at 190° celcius for about ½ hour or until soft, sweet and the outsides have caramelised slightly. Leave to cool.

Roast the pine nuts by placing them in a shallow heavy-based pan. With the heat on medium, toss the pine nuts in the pan until they are a golden colour. Leave to cool.

Assemble all the other salad ingredients in a large bowl and toss. Add the cooled pumpkin and pine nuts. Serve drizzled with Honey Mustard Dressing (see page 60).

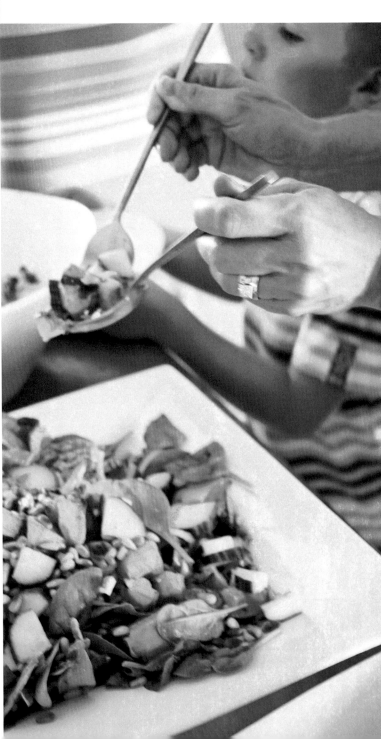

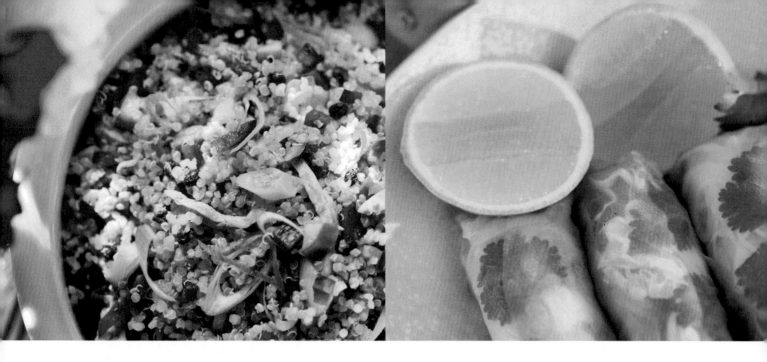

quinoa, cranberry & chicken salad

1 cup quinoa
2 cups water
½ cup dried cranberries
¼ cup currants
¼ cup raw pistachios, shelled
1 small red capsicum, finely chopped
2 spring onions, finely chopped
½ cup parsley, finely chopped
1 cup cucumber, finely diced
1 cooked chicken breast, cut into small cubes
   or thin strips

Bring the quinoa and water to the boil then turn the heat down to low. With the lid on, cook the quinoa until soft and there is no moisture left. Cool then add all other ingredients and mix well.

Delicious served with Spicy Orange Dressing (see page 60). This salad is great for BBQs, picnics or lunchboxes. Makes 4 individual lunch portions.

Rice Paper Rolls are also yummy in lunchboxes. They can have any filling really. I use chicken in place of prawns when I make them for the children's school lunches. I separate the rolls with baking paper so they don't stick together and I make sure the sauce container seals well so it doesn't leak through their lunchbox. To get maximum punch from your sauce, bite the end off the roll and drizzle the sauce into the top of the roll as you eat it. Mmmmmm.

rice paper rolls

50 g dry rice vermicelli (soaked for 10 mins
   in boiling water then drained)
1 cup bean sprouts
½ cup fresh coriander
½ cup carrot, grated
½ cup spring onion, finely sliced
1 cup Asian cabbage, very finely sliced
6 small rice paper sheets
6 large fresh prawns, cooked, peeled and sliced
   in half lengthways

Arrange all the ingredients in a production line in front of you. In a wide, shallow bowl of hot water, immerse one of the rice paper sheets for about 1 minute or until pliable but not soggy. Spread the rice paper sheet in front of you and arrange about a teaspoonful (more or less to taste) of each ingredient, plus the 2 halves of each prawn, along the middle of the rice paper sheet. Fold the top of the sheet over the ingredients then fold each end in towards the middle. Roll up as tightly as you can without breaking the rice paper roll. Repeat this process to make the other rolls.

SAUCE
¼ cup tamari
1 tbsp honey, warmed
½ tsp each of grated ginger and crushed garlic
1 tsp fresh lime juice
A sprinkle of chilli flakes (optional)

Mix the sauce ingredients together and serve in a small bowl alongside the rolls.

main meals

In choosing the meals for this section, I tried to include family favourites so the main meal of the day remained familiar. It was no small feat as many of these meals, such as the Italian-style dishes and the crumbed foods, traditionally rely on wheat ingredients. Plates are scraped clean when these alternative dishes are served at our house so I guess that means they get the thumbs up. I also love sharing the Mint and Cranberry Crusted Lamb dish with family and friends - it's one of our special occasion meals.

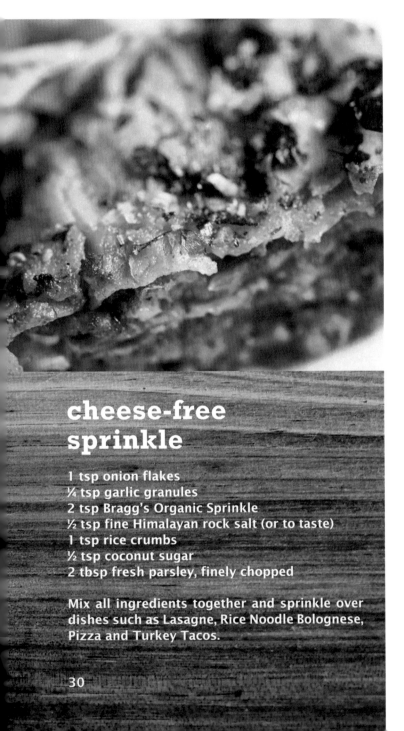

cheese-free sprinkle

1 tsp onion flakes
¼ tsp garlic granules
2 tsp Bragg's Organic Sprinkle
½ tsp fine Himalayan rock salt (or to taste)
1 tsp rice crumbs
½ tsp coconut sugar
2 tbsp fresh parsley, finely chopped

Mix all ingredients together and sprinkle over dishes such as Lasagne, Rice Noodle Bolognese, Pizza and Turkey Tacos.

round deep dish lasagne

1 quantity of Rice Noodle Bolognese (see page 31)
9-12 large round rice paper sheets
Béchamel Sauce
Cheese-free Sprinkle

BÉCHAMEL SAUCE
2 ½ tbsp Nuttelex
2 ½ tbsp cornflour
2 cups rice milk
½ tsp fine Himalayan rock salt
½ tsp gluten-free mustard powder

Melt the Nuttelex in a small saucepan over a medium heat. Mix a little of the rice milk with the cornflour in a small bowl and stir until there are no lumps. Add to the melted Nuttelex and whisk, then add the rest of the rice milk and stir or whisk to combine. Add the other ingredients and continue mixing until the sauce is thick.

In a medium-sized round deep dish, layer each of the lasagne ingredients. Start with a layer of bolognese, then 3 rice paper sheets together, topped with a thin layer of sauce. Repeat this process then finish with a good layer of Béchamel Sauce and Cheese-free Sprinkle on the very top.

Cover with foil and bake at 170° celcius for 20 minutes. Uncover and bake for a further 40 minutes. Serves 4-6.

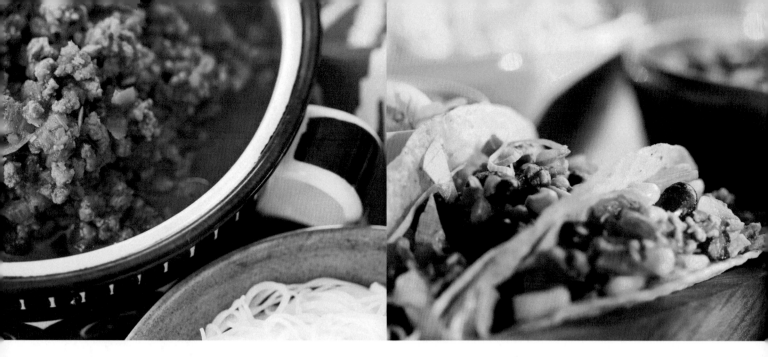

rice noodle bolognese

3 tbsp extra-virgin olive oil
300 g onion, finely chopped
3 large garlic cloves, finely chopped
1 kg beef mince (turkey and lamb are good too)
3 tsp fine Himalayan rock salt
1 tbsp additive-free tomato paste
1 carrot, finely chopped or processed
1 zucchini, finely chopped or processed
1 celery stick, finely chopped or processed
2 x 400 g tins chopped tomatoes
1 tsp cayenne pepper
1 tbsp mixed dried herbs
2 tbsp Braggs All Purpose Seasoning
1 tbsp honey

200 g dry rice vermicelli (fine rice noodles)

Heat the oil in a large heavy-based frying pan and add the onion. Cook over a medium heat until the onion is soft. Add the mince and brown, making sure to break up the mince as it cooks. Add the rest of the ingredients and mix well. Simmer with the lid on for about ½ hour, then continue to simmer with the lid off until half of the juices have been reduced.

In a large saucepan of boiling salted water, add the rice vermicelli and cook for a few minutes until soft. Drain well and serve topped with the bolognese and Cheese-free Sprinkle (see page 30). Serves 4-6.

For a vegetarian bolognese you can substitute the meat for 2 x 400 g tins of brown lentils.

turkey tacos

MINCE MIX
½ kg turkey mince (beef mince is good too)
1 medium onion, finely chopped
1 tbsp extra-virgin olive oil
400 g tin diced tomatoes
400 g tin red kidney beans
⅓ cup corn kernels, fresh or frozen
⅓ cup red capsicum, diced
1 tbsp honey
Cracked black pepper
½ tsp chilli powder (or to taste)
1 tsp fine Himalayan rock salt

ACCOMPANIMENTS
2 cups iceberg lettuce, chopped
2 avocados, mashed or sliced
½ cup spring onion, finely sliced
½ cup cucumber, chopped
1 box of taco shells (approx. 20)

Heat oil in a heavy-based saucepan and fry onion until translucent and soft. Add the meat and stir until browned and fine. Add all other ingredients for the mince mix and stir intermittently until the moisture has reduced and the mixture is firm.

Spread the taco shells on a baking tray and heat for 10 minutes in a preheated 180° celcius oven. Prepare the accompaniments and place them in separate bowls. Take the tacos from the oven and arrange everything on the table for self-service. Serves 5-6.

We love Turkey Taco night!

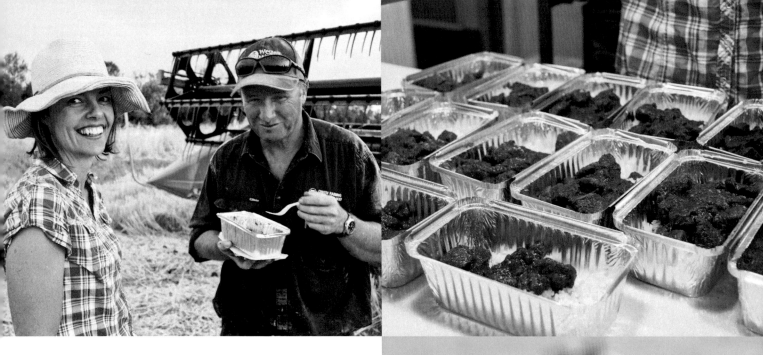

sweet beef curry

1 kg beef (casserole steak), cubed
2 tbsp coconut oil
1 large onion, finely chopped
1 apple, peeled and chopped
1 tbsp organic curry powder
1 tsp ground fennel
1 tsp cardamom seeds
1 tsp caraway seeds
5 whole cloves
1 tsp fine Himalayan rock salt
2 ripe bananas, peeled and chopped
½ cup sultanas
2 cups water
2 tbsp Braggs All Purpose Seasoning
1 heaped tbsp arrowroot mixed with a little water

Heat oil on high in a large heavy-based casserole dish. Quickly brown beef in batches and set aside. Add onions and apple to the casserole dish and cook over medium heat until soft. Stir in curry and other spices then add all other ingredients (except the arrowroot mixture) and combine.

Place lid on casserole dish and cook in the oven at 160° celcius for 2½ hours or until the meat is tender. Stir through the arrowroot mixture until sauce thickens. Serve with brown rice. Makes 5-6 portions.

For extra tenderness and flavour, I recommend making this curry the day before eating. It's a great dish to satisfy a hungry family or a team of workers.

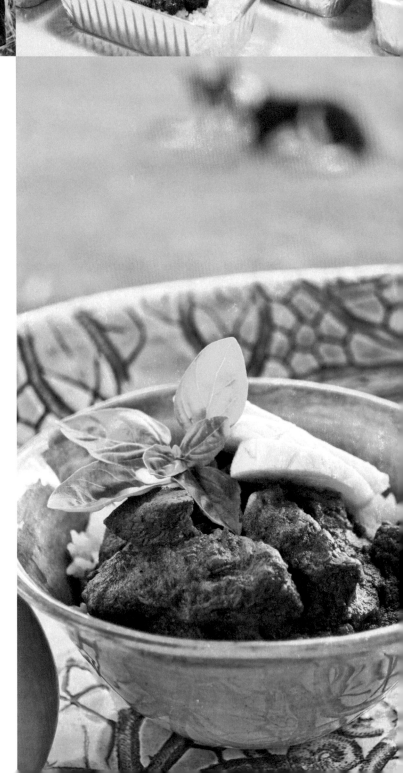

chicken nuggets

This recipe was inspired by Jamie Oliver's 'Food Revolution' cooking series. I love what Jamie has done for so many families and institutions. I'm a huge fan of his and I'm sure he will save lives through his healthy food education.

1 whole chicken breast
2 cups approx. rice crumbs
A dish of warm water
1 tsp lemon zest
1 garlic clove, crushed
1 tbsp parsley, finely chopped
Coconut oil for shallow frying
Fine Himalayan rock salt to taste
Cracked black pepper

Separate chicken breast into 2 and cut in half widthways. Then cut each ¼ breast into 3 lengths, so 12 lengths in total. Heat a heavy-based frying pan with enough oil to cover the base of the pan. Mix the rice crumbs, garlic, parsley, lemon zest, salt and pepper on a flat plate. Individually dip the chicken pieces into the dish of warm water then roll in the rice crumb mix.

Fry the chicken on each side until golden brown, then drain on absorbent paper. Serve with sweet potato mash and a crisp green salad. Makes 4 portions.

barra fish fingers

Any fish can be used for these fish fingers just so long as it doesn't have delicate flesh. I love the flavour of barramundi fillets and their flesh holds together well when crumbed and fried. 'Barra' is also the name of the property I grew up on and I have fond memories of fishing there as a child!

2-3 barramundi fillets, cut into thick fingers

Use the chicken nuggets rice crumb mix above and follow the same directions for crumbing and frying. Serve with homemade sweet potato wedges. Makes 4-5 portions.

Delicious with Caper & Dill Sauce (see page 60).

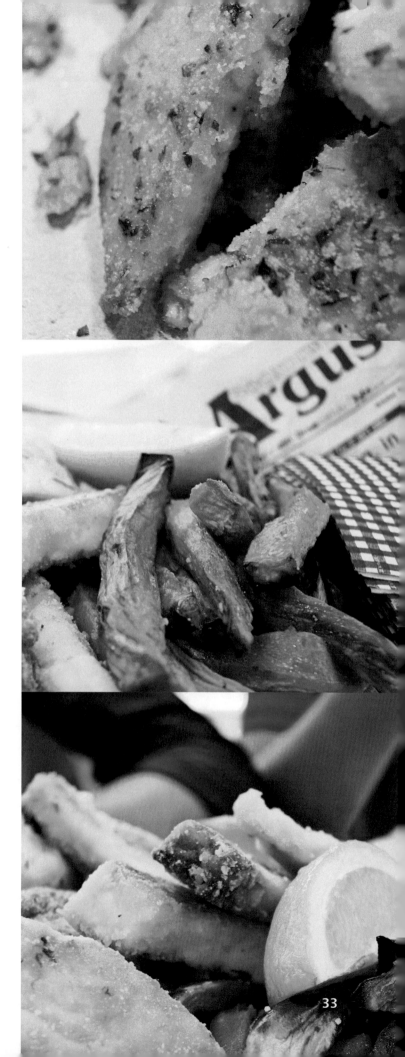

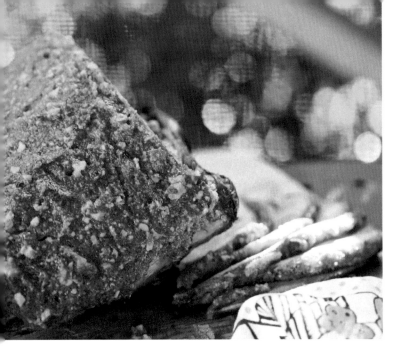

orange, mustard & nut-glazed ham

4 kg approx. leg of ham (salted only)
2 x 285 g jars Dick Smith's Marmalade
1 tbsp coconut sugar
80 g walnuts, crumbled
50 g rice crumbs
2 tsp water
1 tsp extra-virgin olive oil
1 tsp cracked black pepper
1 tsp fine Himalayan rock salt
½ tsp chilli flakes

Place an old plate in the bottom of a large boiling pot to prevent the ham sticking to the bottom. Put ham in and fill with water to cover the main body of the ham, don't worry if the end is sticking out. Bring the water to boil and leave boiling for about ½ hour. Remove and place ham on a cutting board. Gently peel the skin off using a knife if necessary. Diamond score the fat left covering the ham. Bake at 175° celcius for 15 minutes to open up the diamond shapes in the fat.

Combine the marmalade, coconut sugar, walnuts, rice crumbs, cracked pepper, salt, water, oil and chilli flakes to make the glaze. Press half of this glaze mixture all over the leg and bake for 25 minutes at 175° celcius. Add the remainder of the glaze and bake again at 175° celcius for another 25 minutes. Let the ham stand for ½ hour. Then carve and serve with vegetables or salad. Will satisfy a large crowd.

miranda kerr's slow roasted chicken

Since finding this delicious recipe on Miranda Kerr's website, koraorganics.com, our whole family has enthusiastically tucked into this dish on a regular basis. I love the fact that it's quick to prepare and I can pop it in the oven before the kid's footy training or swimming club and come home to a ready-made delectable dish.

1 organic free-range chicken
3 onions, peeled and quartered
6 garlic cloves, peeled
3 tbsp coconut oil
3 tsp Braggs All Purpose Seasoning
Juice of 1 lemon
½ tsp fine Himalayan rock salt
¼ tsp turmeric
1 sprig of rosemary, chopped (or 2 tsp dried)

Wash the chicken and lie it breast down in a roasting dish (that has a lid). Place the onion and garlic around the chicken and in the cavity. Spoon the coconut oil onto the chicken and spread. Pour the Braggs seasoning and lemon juice over the chicken and finally sprinkle with salt, turmeric and rosemary. Place the lid on the roasting dish and cook in the oven covered for 3½ hours at 140° celcius. Baste the chicken with the juices every hour if possible. Take the lid off and continue to bake for another ½ hour to brown the chicken. Serve with roasted vegetables. Makes 5-6 portions.

All the left over onions and juices are used as the stock in the Zesty Carrot Soup (see page 24).

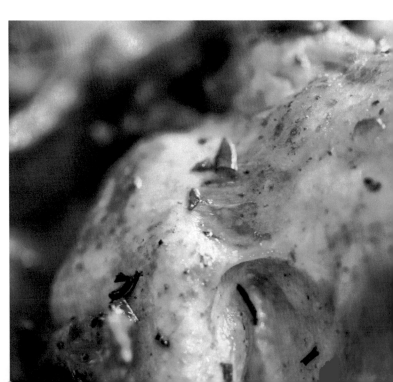

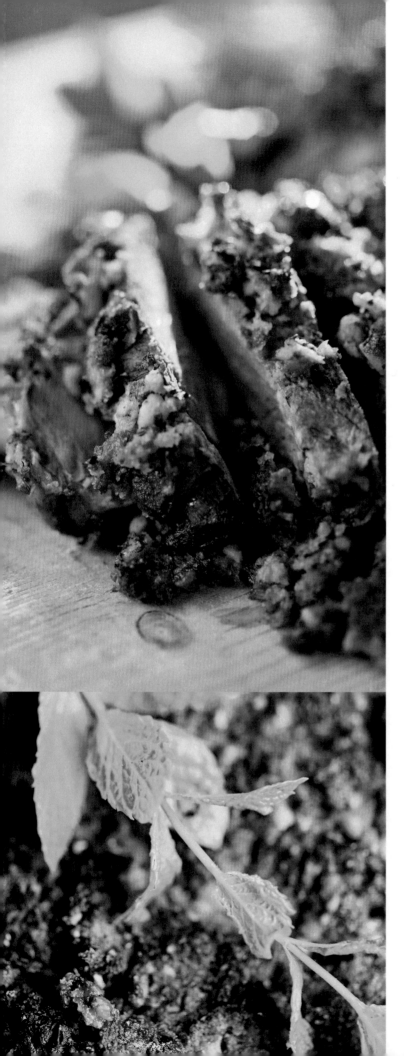

mint & cranberry crusted lamb

2 kg approx. leg of lamb, deboned and evenly
    butterflied (ask your butcher to do this)
1 onion, peeled and quartered
3 garlic cloves
⅓ cup fresh parsley (tightly packed)
⅓ cup fresh mint (tightly packed)
⅓ cup raw cashews
½ cup dried cranberries
⅓ cup rice crumbs
1 tsp fine Himalayan rock salt
1 tsp fresh rosemary, chopped (or 2 tsp dried)
½ tsp ground cumin
½ tsp ground coriander
1 tbsp extra-virgin olive oil
½ tsp cracked black pepper
1 tbsp honey
2 tbsp water

Process the onion, garlic, herbs, cashews and
cranberries until finely chopped. Transfer to a
bowl and mix with the other ingredients. Drizzle
a little oil in the base of a large baking dish and
place the butterflied lamb, skin side down, into
the dish. Spread the herb mix over the top of the
leg. Drizzle a little more oil and sprinkle some
more salt over the dish. Bake for ½ hour at 180°
celcius. Then continue to bake at 165° celcius for
a further 1½ hours for well-done meat. Serves 6
with leftovers.

*Beautiful as a cold meat with no need for relish,
as the onions, herbs and cranberries amalgamate
with the meat juices to make a gorgeous 'jammy'
addition to the lamb, hot or cold.*

*As a child, I grew up eating lamb, hogget and a
lot of mutton. I loved it all then and still do now. I
created this recipe as a tribute to good grass-fed
lamb. It has all the complementary ingredients I
love in a meat dish - a bit of tang, some sweetness,
good salt and fresh herbs, yum!*

*In Australia, generally lamb refers to all meat
from a sheep under one year. Hogget is over a
year and mutton is meat from an adult sheep.
This dish is also great using hogget, you may need
to pre-order it from your butcher though as lamb
is more popular nowadays.*

Nibbles, dips & Crackers

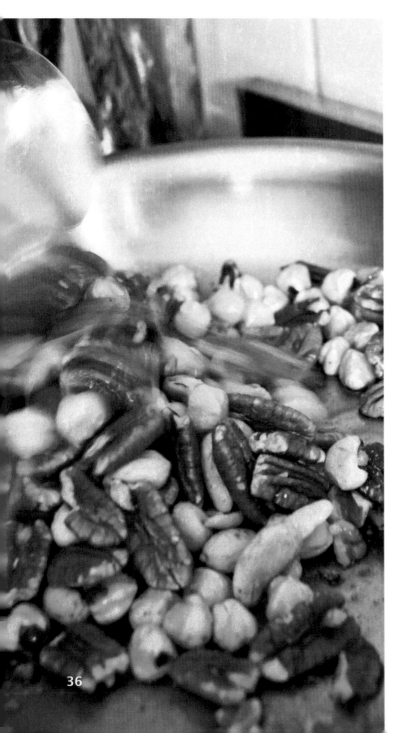

salted & roasted nuts

1 cup mixed raw unsalted nuts (cashews, pecan
    nuts, hazelnuts, peanuts or walnuts)
Extra-virgin olive oil for roasting nuts
Fine Himalayan rock salt to taste

Drizzle oil over the bottom of a small heavy-based
pan and add the nuts. Over a medium to hot heat,
shake and toss the nuts for about 4 minutes. Tip
the hot nuts in a bowl and sprinkle with salt and
toss again.

*The nuts will harden and crisp up as they cool. If
you find the salt not sticking to the nuts add a tiny
bit more oil and toss again.*

popcorn

¾ cup popping corn
2 tbsp extra-virgin olive oil
1 tsp fine Himalayan rock salt (or to taste)

In a heavy-based pan with a lid, add 1 tablespoon
of the oil and the popping corn. Mix a little to coat
the corn with the oil, then level out across the pan.
Turn the heat to high and place the lid on the pan.

Listen for the popping and when it slows to only a
couple of pops every couple of seconds, take the
pan from the heat. Tip the popcorn into a large
bowl, drizzle with remaining oil and sprinkle with
salt. Toss well.

Something that made giving up alcohol easier, was keeping up the little ritual of some savoury nibbles at the end of the day. Having some nibbles on hand also staves off any hunger pains while dinner is being prepared. My husband loves the roasted nuts and popcorn is a family favourite. I mix up my choices, although I do adore hommus with crackers and veggie sticks.

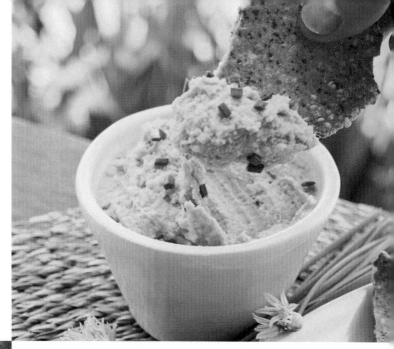

hommus

250 g chickpeas, soft-boiled or tinned
  (drained and liquid reserved)
¼ cup extra-virgin olive oil
½ tsp fine Himalayan rock salt
2 tbsp tahini
1 tbsp fresh lemon juice
2 tsp ground cumin
1 garlic clove, crushed (add more if desired)
Fresh herbs and extra-virgin olive oil for serving

Blend all ingredients until smooth. If the mix is a bit too stiff, add a little of the reserved chickpea water. The flavour of hommus improves when it is covered and left in the fridge overnight. To serve, drizzle with extra-virgin olive oil and sprinkle with fresh herbs or paprika.

When I have time to prepare a selection of nibbles for weekend get-togethers or special occasions, I find hommus is lovely served with Helen's Crispy Seed Crackers (see page 38).

I also love to serve a big bowl of hommus to my kids for afternoon tea accompanied by a great selection of raw vegetable sticks, including carrot, celery, zucchini, broccoli and cauliflower. I find this is a great snack which keeps them going until dinner time. Hommus is easy to make and it's something my daughter has enjoyed making since she was about six years old.

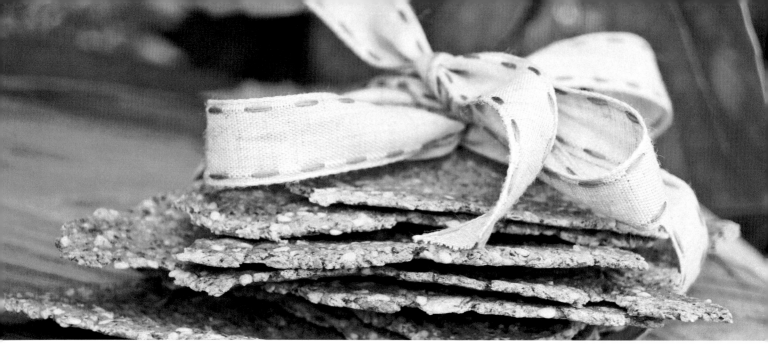

helen's crispy seed crackers

¼ cup seeds (you can use a mixture of poppy, sunflower, pepita, sesame or chia seeds)
¼ cup water
½ cup buckwheat flour
1 tsp yellow mustard seeds
1 tsp mixed dry herbs
1 tsp ground cumin
1 tsp fine Himalayan rock salt
¼ tsp cracked black pepper

Soak seeds for 2 hours in water. Combine the seeds and water in a food processor and process. Add the remaining ingredients and continue to process until mixture binds into a dough, adding a little more water if necessary. Preheat the oven to 175° celcius. Roll the dough into a ball then between 2 sheets of baking paper, roll the dough out until approximately 2 mm thick. Remove the top piece of baking paper and transfer to a lightly oiled baking tray by flipping the flattened dough over and peeling the remaining paper off. Bake as 1 large cracker for approximately 25-30 minutes or until brown and crisp. Cool and break into rustic pieces to serve with your favourite dip.

My sister-in-law Helen created this recipe for crackers to have with her lunch at work. I've adapted it a little and for extra yumminess, I recommend sprinkling a beautiful artisan flake salt on the top before baking. For a special occasion, use a pasta cutter to create fancy-edged crackers.

dukka

60 g sunflower seeds
40 g sesame seeds
1 tbsp coriander seeds
1 tbsp cumin seeds
1 tbsp dried onion flakes
1 tsp cracked black pepper
1 tsp flake salt (Murray River, Cyprus or Maldon)

Preheat oven to 180° celcius. On a baking tray, spread the sunflower seeds and sesame seeds. Bake for approximately 4 minutes then toss and turn the mix. Bake for a further 4 minutes. Set aside to cool.

Dry roast the coriander and cumin seeds in a frying pan until aromatic and slightly golden. Pour all the seeds into a food processor and process until crumbed. Transfer to a bowl and add all other ingredients. Mix well and store in an airtight container. Serve with dips and crackers or on toasted gluten-free bread drizzled with extra-virgin olive oil. (See pages 40 and 41 for bread recipes).

carrot & coriander dip

400 g carrot, grated
½ cup approx. water
1 tbsp Braggs All Purpose Seasoning
1 tsp apple cider vinegar
1 tsp extra-virgin olive oil (add more if needed)
1 tsp ground cumin
1 tsp ground coriander
½ tsp fresh oregano, finely chopped (1 tsp dried)
1 garlic clove, crushed
Fine Himalayan rock salt to taste
Cracked black pepper
Fresh coriander, chopped for garnish

Simmer carrot in water with Braggs seasoning until soft. Then purée with all the remaining ingredients, keeping the coriander to garnish.

beetroot dip

1 large beetroot, peeled, cubed and boiled
  in salted water until soft
40 g silken tofu
2 tbsp tahini
2 tbsp extra-virgin olive oil
1 garlic clove, crushed
1 tsp fresh lemon juice
½ tbsp fresh dill, chopped (and some to garnish)
¼ tsp fine Himalayan rock salt
Cracked black pepper

Blend ingredients until smooth. Garnish with dill.

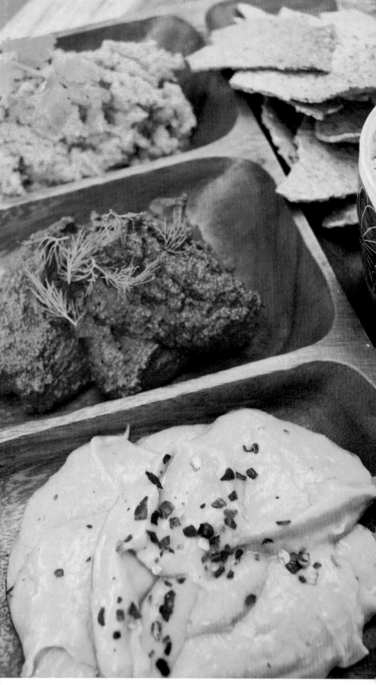

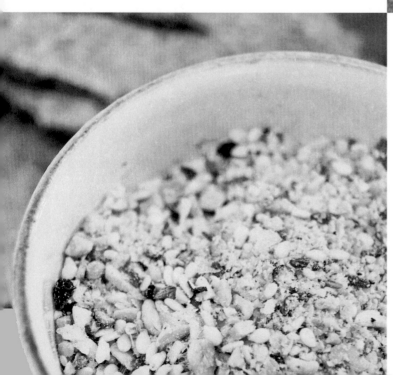

avocado & sweet chilli dip

Flesh of 1 avocado
1 garlic clove, crushed
30 g silken tofu
1 tbsp maple syrup
¼ tsp fine Himalayan rock salt
Pinch of chilli powder
Chilli flakes to garnish

Purée all ingredients together and garnish with chilli flakes.

BreaDs & Loaves

farmer's fruit & nut loaf

2 cups dried fruit (a combination of raisins,
 dates, apricots, figs or whatever you have
 in the cupboard - chop the larger fruit)
1 cup hot water
1 cup gluten-free self-raising flour
1 tsp xanthan gum
½ cup almond meal
¼ cup quinoa flakes
½ tsp mixed spice
½ cup walnuts, crumbled
3 tbsp macadamia oil
½ tsp fine Himalayan rock salt
Pepitas and sunflower seeds for decoration

Soak the dried fruit in the hot water for at least
½ hour. Preheat oven to 170° celcius. Line a
standard-sized loaf tin with baking paper. Drain
the fruit and reserve the water. Mix all ingredients
together and add the reserved water as necessary
to make a firm dough.

Spoon the dough into the loaf tin. Sprinkle top
with pepitas and sunflower seeds and press down
into the dough. Bake for approximately 1 hour
until the loaf is golden brown, the top is firm to
touch and a skewer comes out clean.

*This wholesome, hearty, country loaf is a tribute
to farmers everywhere! Great served warm with a
spread of Nuttelex at smoko time.*

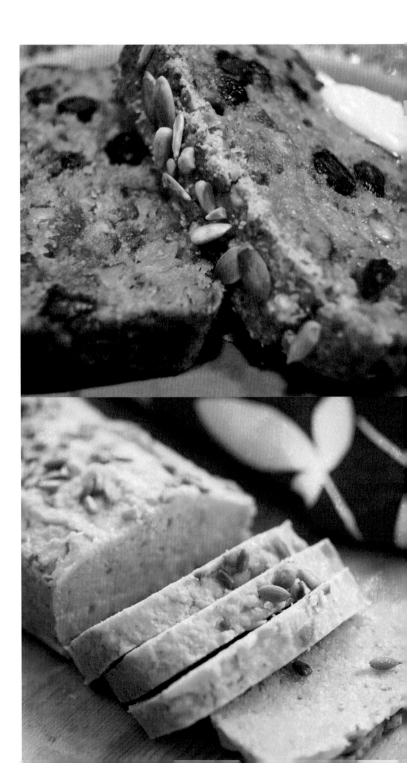

Nailing a good gluten-free bread recipe has been important in order for me to completely eliminate gluten from my household. Everyone in our house enjoys pizza on a Friday night, so a great gluten-free pizza is another important staple for us and for many other families I'm sure. I have included the tastiest toppings I could think of to compensate for the no-cheese pizza.

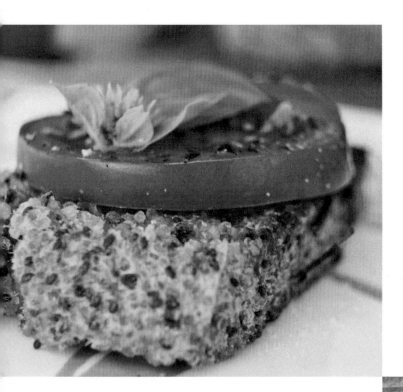

teresa cutter's gluten-free bread

Adapted from one of Teresa Cutter's great gluten-free recipes on her website, thehealthychef.com.

600 g quinoa seeds, whole and uncooked
1 ½ cups water (and extra for soaking quinoa)
60 g chia seeds
¼ cup extra-virgin olive oil
1 tsp bicarb soda
1 tsp fine Himalayan rock salt
Juice of ½ a lemon
1 tbsp fresh rosemary, chopped (optional)

Soak quinoa in plenty of cold water overnight in the fridge. Soak chia seeds in ½ cup of the water until gel-like, stir before using. Drain the quinoa and rinse well through a strainer. Place the quinoa into a food processor. Add chia gel, 1 cup of water, olive oil, bicarb soda, sea salt and lemon juice. Add rosemary now if you choose. Process until combined and mixture is thick.

Spoon into a large loaf tin lined with baking paper. Bake for 1-1½ hours at 160° celcius or until firm to touch. Remove from the tin and cool completely. The bread should be slightly moist in the middle and not overcooked. Slice and serve when cold, cutting with a serrated knife. Can be stored in the fridge for up to 1 week or frozen for up to 3 months.

Use whole quinoa not rolled. Hulled millet can also be used in place of the quinoa.

nutty cornbread

⅓ cup almond meal
⅓ cup polenta
⅓ cup rice crumbs
1 cup gluten-free self-raising flour
1 cup rice milk
2 tbsp extra-virgin olive oil
1 large apple or pear, peeled and grated
½ tsp fine Himalayan rock salt
1 tbsp seeds to sprinkle on top before cooking

Combine all ingredients and pour into a small loaf tin. Bake at 170° celcius for 40-45 minutes.

serving suggestions for these breads

- Lightly toasted and topped with fresh sliced tomato, drizzled with extra-virgin olive oil and sprinkled with fine Himalayan rock salt.
- Lightly toasted and dipped in your favourite winter soup (see page 24 and 25).
- Lightly toasted and spread with Nuttelex and sugar-free jam or marmalade.
- Lightly toasted and topped with nut butter, sliced banana and a drizzle of honey.
- To use as a healthy pizza base – bake as a flat bread instead of a loaf.

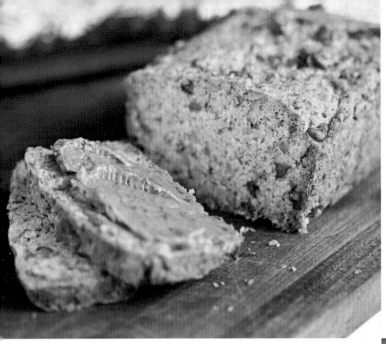

pizza dough

2 cups gluten-free self-raising flour
2 tsp xanthan gum
2 tsp fine Himalayan rock salt
2 tbsp extra-virgin olive oil
¾ cup water
Sprinkling of flour mixed with polenta for rolling
A large pizza baking tray generously oiled with
  extra-virgin olive oil

Preheat the oven to 220° celcius on the grill setting and place a rack closest to the grill. Whisk the flour and xanthan gum together. Add all other ingredients and mix well. Leave covered in a bowl for about ¼ hour.

banana bread with orange spread

300 g banana, mashed
50 g Nuttelex, melted
2 tbsp coconut oil, melted
1 tbsp honey
¼ cup coconut sugar
1 ½ cups gluten-free self-raising flour
1 tsp xanthan gum
1 tsp cinnamon
¼ cup ground nut meal
½ cup walnuts, crumbled
1 tsp fine Himalayan rock salt

Combine all ingredients well. Spoon and level into a small lined loaf tin. Bake in a 170° celcius oven for 35-40 minutes. Cool on a wire rack.

CHOCOLATE BANANA BREAD OR CAKE
To create a lovely rich chocolate banana bread or cake, add ¼ cup raw cacao powder and 1 tablespoon of water to the recipe above. Can be baked in a loaf tin or a round cake tin.

MIMI'S ORANGE SPREAD
2 tbsp Nuttelex
1 tbsp coconut sugar
1 tsp orange zest
1 tsp fresh orange juice

Mix all ingredients and spread on thick slices of the banana bread loaf.

My daughter Mimi adapted this Junior Masterchef recipe especially for my last Mother's Day brekky.

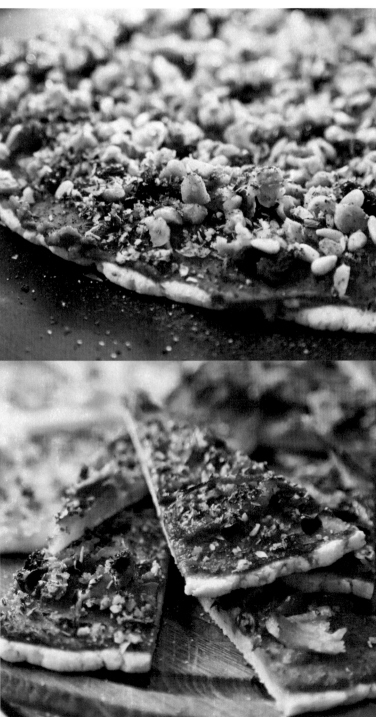

Spread a large sheet of baking paper on a flat surface and sprinkle with polenta. Divide the dough in half, placing one dough ball back in the covered bowl. Place the other on the baking paper and using a rolling pin, roll out the pizza dough into a flat round disc about ½ cm thick (a little smaller in diameter than the pizza baking tray that you will be using).

When you are happy with the size of your base, transfer it to the pizza tray. This is easier if you put the pizza tray on top of the base and flip it over onto the tray, then peel off the baking paper. If it sticks to the paper, use more polenta and flour to roll with next time.

Place pizza base under grill for approximately 3-4 minutes or until light brown. Watch while the pizza base cooks as it does burn quickly. Take the tray out and using a large egg flip, flip over the pizza base and repeat the grilling process for the other side. Take the base out of the oven and apply the toppings. Grill until toppings are hot and bubbling. Repeat the entire process using the second dough ball.

pizza toppings

1. Spread Onion Jam (see page 58) over pizza base and sprinkle with 1 teaspoon of finely chopped fresh rosemary and Cheese-free Sprinkle (see page 30). This pizza makes a great appetiser.

2. Generously spread Tomato Sauce (see page 59) over pizza base. Add ¼ cup of chopped olives, 1 tablespoon of chopped salted anchovies, ¼ cup of finely sliced capsicum, ⅓ cup of sliced nitrate-free ham pieces, 1 teaspoon of chopped fresh thyme, a drizzle of extra-virgin olive oil and top with Cheese-free Sprinkle.

3. Spread 2 crushed garlic cloves over pizza base. Drizzle with extra-virgin olive oil and top with Cheese-free Sprinkle.

4. Spread ½ cup of mashed roasted pumpkin or sweet potato over pizza base. Add 1 teaspoon of chopped fresh sage, ¼ cup of raisins (soaked for 2 hours in 2 tablespoons of apple cider vinegar and drained well), ½ teaspoon of ground nutmeg, 2 tablespoons of chopped tinned chickpeas, 1 tablespoon of pine nuts, a pinch of cayenne pepper, a drizzle of extra-virgin olive oil and top with Cheese-free Sprinkle.

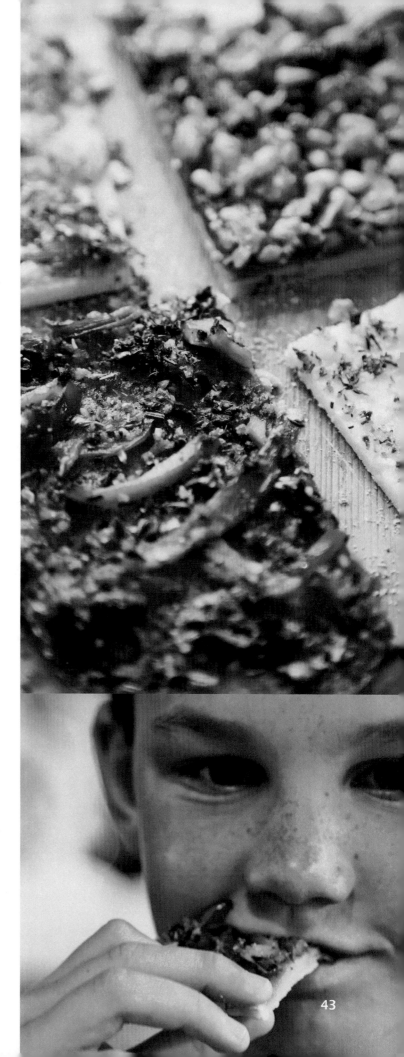

Cakes, Bars & Biscuits

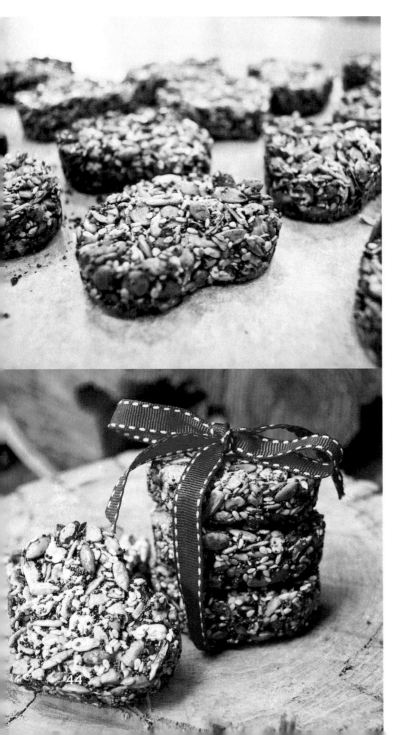

budgie snacks

1 cup pepitas
1 cup sunflower seeds
½ cup poppy seeds
½ cup sesame seeds
1 tbsp chia seeds
1 tsp flaxseeds (optional)
½ cup walnuts, crumbled or chopped
1 cup puffed millet
½ tsp ground cinnamon
½ tsp fine Himalayan rock salt
½ cup honey, warmed

Stir all ingredients together until combined. Press a 1 cm thick layer into shallow, lined baking tins of various shapes. Alternatively, press the mixture into 1 large tray to break into pieces when cooked. Bake in oven at approximately 170° celcius for about 25 minutes, then turn oven off and leave snacks inside to cool and crisp. Store in an airtight container.

Tip: To press the mixture into the tin, cover it with a sheet of baking paper and press down. You can also use the back of a spoon to press the mixture down (keep wiping the spoon with a damp cloth to prevent sticking).

The heart-shaped Budgie Snacks are great dipped in Honey Chocolate (see page 53).

To create an edible decoration to hang on the Christmas tree, make a hole approximately 5 mm in diameter with the end of a chopstick before the Budgie Snacks are put in the oven. You can thread ribbon through the hole once they have been baked and are cool.

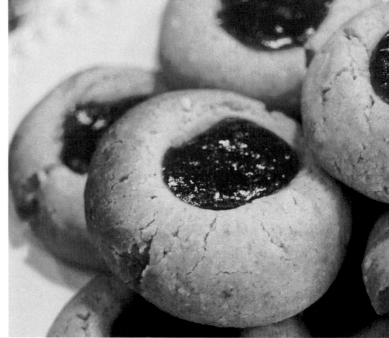

Cakes, bars and biscuits were the first recipes I started converting as they were the foods I knew I couldn't go without. Being a country girl, smoko has always been an integral part of my day and I like nothing more than a little treat with my hot cuppa. For me it was important that I wasn't 'missing out' when everyone else was tucking into their wheaty, dairy-laden morning tea.

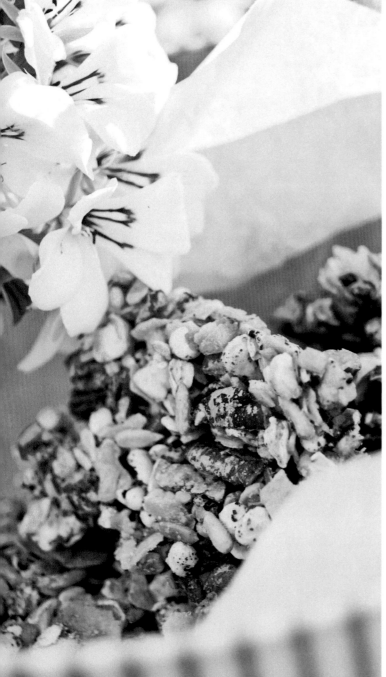

jam drops

1 cup besan (chickpea) flour
1 cup buckwheat flour
1 ½ cups almond meal
½ tsp fine Himalayan rock salt
½ tsp ground cinnamon
½ cup macadamia oil
½ cup maple syrup
Dick Smith's Magnificent Jam

Preheat oven to 180° celcius. In a bowl, combine all ingredients except the jam to make a firm dough. Form walnut-sized balls from this biscuit dough and place evenly on lined baking trays. Make a small depression in each ball and fill with jam. Bake for 15 minutes or until golden brown. Allow to cool and store airtight. Makes approximately 30.

Inspired by 'Lalo's Famous Cookie' recipe in Gwyneth Paltrow's book 'Notes From My Kitchen Table', published by Boxtree Limited.

pecan puff bars

2 cups puffed buckwheat
1 cup pecans, coarsely chopped
½ cup sunflower seeds
¾ cup flaked coconut or ½ cup desiccated
½ tsp fine Himalayan rock salt
½ cup maple syrup
3 tbsp tahini

Mix all the ingredients and press into a lined shallow slice tin approximately 18 cm x 28 cm. Bake at 150° celcius for approximately 30 minutes. Cool in the tin then break into pieces. Store in an airtight container.

If you are after a celebratory cake for a birthday, christening or even a wedding, then baking this gorgeous cake means you don't have to miss out on a treat during that special occasion.

I absolutely adore spiced fruit cakes but many leave me with uncomfortable heartburn. I was so happy when I created this cake as it is more gentle on my stomach. One of the secrets is to use sulphite-free dried fruit. Be mindful though, there is still a lot of fruit sugar in this recipe so enjoy a slice only every now and then.

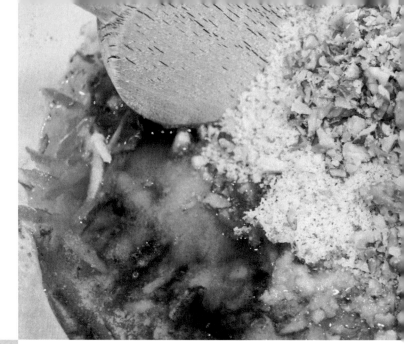

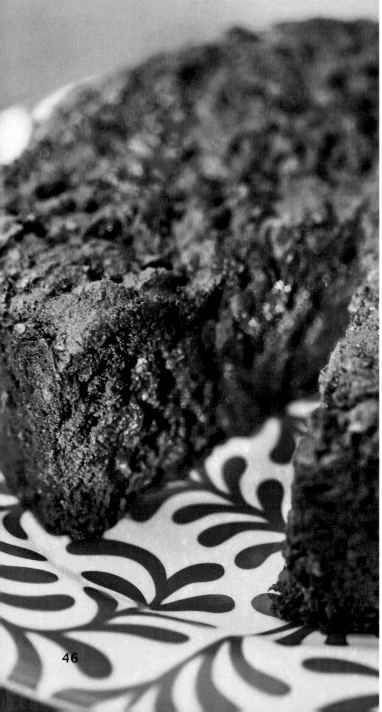

rich spiced fruit cake

250 g sultanas
250 g dried fruit (a combination of dates, cranberries, prunes, raisins, currants, figs, pear, apple and apricots - chop the larger fruit)
50 g goji berries
20 g flaxseeds
350 ml water
1 tbsp orange juice
1 tbsp orange zest
65 g macadamia oil
1 tbsp pomegranate molasses
1 ½ cups garbanzo and fava flour
1 tsp xanthan gum
1 ½ tsp bicarb soda
¼ cup raw cacao powder
55 g coconut sugar
3 tsp mixed spice
1 tsp fine Himalayan rock salt
½ cup blanched almonds, roughly chopped

Soak all fruit and the flaxseeds in the water, juice and zest overnight. Preheat the oven to 140° celcius and line a medium-sized spring-form tin with baking paper. Mix all wet ingredients together. In a separate bowl, sift all dry ingredients (except the almonds). Add dry to wet and mix well. The mix should be thick but if you think it is too dry add a little more water. Add the almonds and combine.

Spoon the mixture into the lined tin and spread evenly, making sure there are no air pockets. Smooth the top of the cake and bake for 1½ hours or until the cake feels firm. Leave in the tin and cool for ½ hour then remove and let the cake cool completely on a rack. Store in an airtight container.

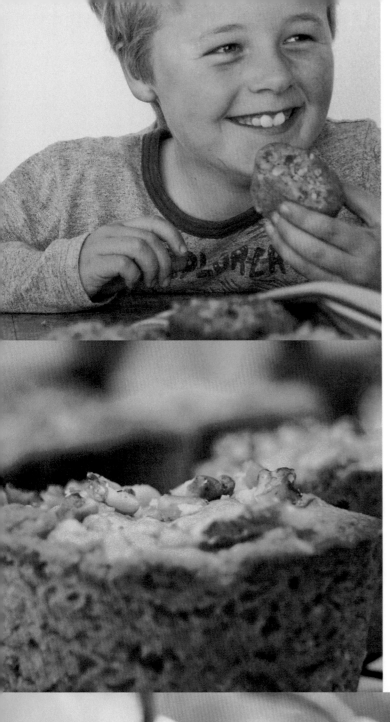

carrot & apple cakes

1 ½ cups gluten-free self-raising flour
½ cup almond meal
1 tsp mixed spice
½ cup olive oil
½ cup honey
½ cup apple, grated
½ cup carrot, grated
½ cup walnuts, crumbled or finely chopped
Extra crumbled walnuts for decoration

Preheat oven to 180° celcius. Combine all the ingredients in a large bowl. Spoon mixture into a standard-sized muffin tray, filling three quarters full. Sprinkle with extra crumbled walnuts. Bake for 20-25 minutes until cakes are golden and spring back when touched. Makes approximately 12.

pear & almond biscuits

2 ½ cups almond meal
1 tsp ground cinnamon
1 tsp fine Himalayan rock salt
½ cup pear, grated
1 tbsp maple syrup
1 tbsp tapioca flour mixed with 1 tbsp water

Mix all ingredients in a bowl to make a dough. Roll spoonfuls of dough into balls and press onto a lined tray. Bake at 170° celcius for 15-20 minutes. Makes approximately 16.

Great biscuits for babies - Maggie loved these!

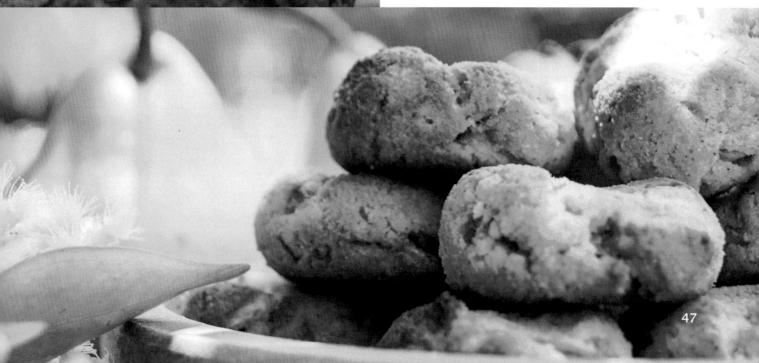

honey joys

I was after some yummy old-fashioned party foods for my kid's birthday parties, so I adapted this popular classic I used to love making as a child.

2 cups gluten-free cornflakes
¼ cup coconut sugar
45 g Nuttelex
1 tbsp honey

Warm the Nuttelex, coconut sugar and honey in a small saucepan until combined. Add to cornflakes and mix well. Spoon into patty cases and bake at 170° celcius for 10 minutes. This mix fills approximately 12 standard patty cases. Alternatively, you can press the mix into a tin to cut into bars or break into pieces once cooked.

I've discovered there are a variety of ingredients that can be used instead of the cornflakes. All variations are equally delish and are gobbled up at kid's get-togethers and parties.

Cornflake alternatives you might like to try:

* 2 cups freshly popped corn
* 2 cups buckwheat puffs
* 2 cups brown rice flakes
* 2 cups puffed rice

You can also add ¼ cup of mixed chopped nuts or seeds to these ingredients. This recipe is great to experiment with, so mix and match ingredients to create your own ideal Honey Joy!

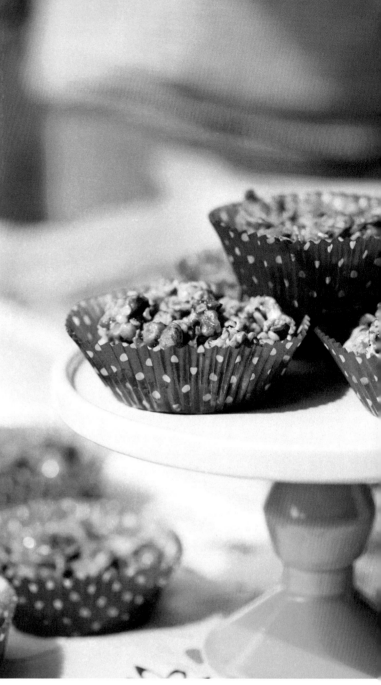

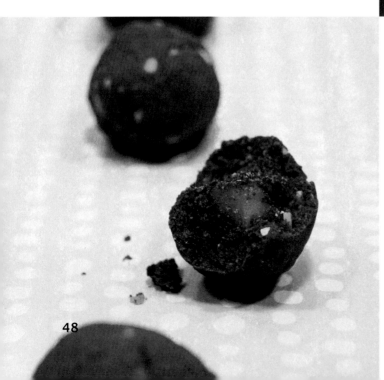

choc walnut balls

1 ½ cups gluten-free plain flour
½ cup desiccated coconut
⅓ cup raw cacao powder
⅓ cup walnuts, chopped
½ cup maple syrup
80 g Nuttelex, melted

Preheat oven to 180° celcius. Mix all ingredients together. Roll mixture into walnut-sized balls. Press onto greased or lined baking trays. Alternatively, roll the mixture into a log and cut into discs. Bake for 15 minutes until a little cracked - they will harden as they cool. Makes approximately 24. Cool and store in an airtight container.

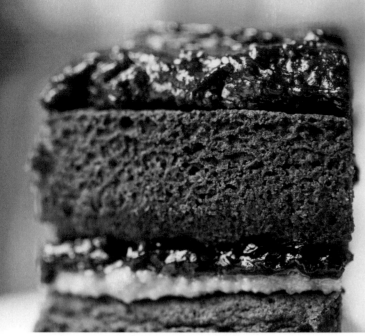

ICING
4 tbsp cashew nut butter
4 tbsp raw cacao powder
4 tbsp maple syrup

Mix the icing ingredients together, adding a little hot water if mix is too stiff. Spread the filling on top of one cake then spread the jam over the filling. Place the other cake on top to sandwich the filling. Spread the icing over the top cake then decorate.

It's important to our family that we have a delicious cake everyone loves for our birthdays, especially when the cake goes to school to be shared with classmates. This rich and decadent cake absolutely fits the bill!

choc layer cake

Adapted from Erin McKenna's German Chocolate Cake recipe from her book 'Babycakes - Covers the Classics' published by Clarkson Potter.

350 g Bob's Red Mill 'All Purpose Baking Flour'
50 g almond meal
1 ½ tbsp baking powder
½ tsp bicarb soda
1 ½ tsp xanthan gum
¼ tsp fine Himalayan rock salt
65 g raw cacao powder
350 ml maple syrup
180 g coconut oil
210 g apple purée
½ cup hot water

Preheat oven to 170° celcius. Line 2 x 23 cm spring-form tins with baking paper and brush the sides with coconut oil. Sift dry ingredients into a large bowl and whisk to combine. Gradually whisk in wet ingredients until a loose batter forms. Pour evenly into the 2 tins. Bake for 15 minutes then rotate the cake tins 180 degrees, swap shelves and bake for a further 20 minutes. Leave in the tins for 5 minutes, then loosen the sides with a knife and turn out onto a rack to cool.

CASHEW CREAM FILLING
100 ml water
1 tbsp coconut sugar
130 g raw cashews

Dissolve coconut sugar in the water then add cashews and soak for at least 2 hours, preferably overnight. Mix in a processor to a smooth paste.

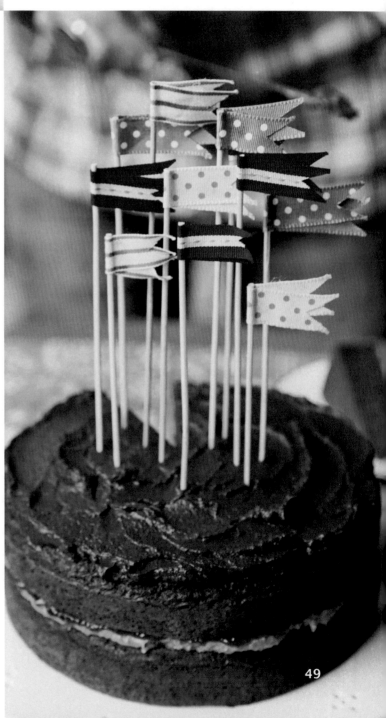

desserts & sweet Treats

chocolate coconut tart

BASE
120 g almond meal
15 pitted dates
½ tsp fine Himalayan rock salt
1 tsp coconut oil

Mix all ingredients in a food processor until the mixture sticks together when pressed between your fingers. Pour into a 20 cm spring-form tin lined with foil. Press mixture evenly across the base of the tin and freeze.

FILLING
250 g avocado
50 g ripe banana
½ cup coconut sugar
½ cup raw cacao powder
50 g coconut oil
¼ tsp fine Himalayan rock salt

Process all ingredients until very smooth. Pour onto the frozen base and spread evenly. Place back in the freezer and take out 15 minutes before serving.

BERRY COULIS (Optional)
2 cups frozen berries
¼ cup maple syrup

Combine and simmer all ingredients over a low heat until the liquid has been reduced by half. Cool and drizzle the coulis over the tart for a decadent slice of heaven!

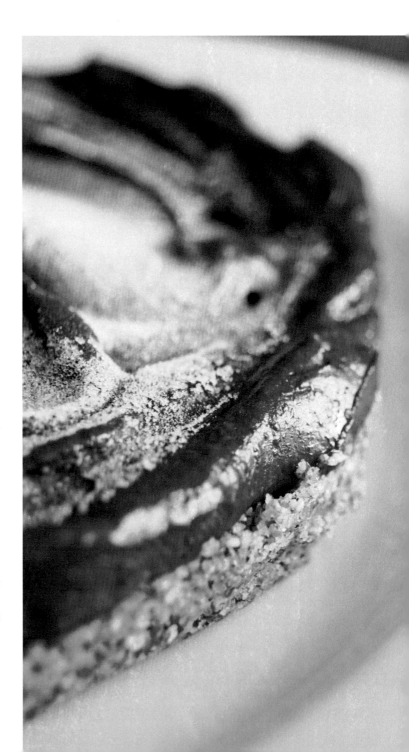

A celebratory or festive meal just wouldn't be the same without ending in dessert, whether it's a little Choc Orange Truffle or a decadent slice of Cashew, Macadamia and Raspberry Tart topped with Berry Crumble. What I love about these desserts, is that there's no uncomfortable 'arggghhh' feeling at the end of the meal. I am mindful though - everything in moderation.

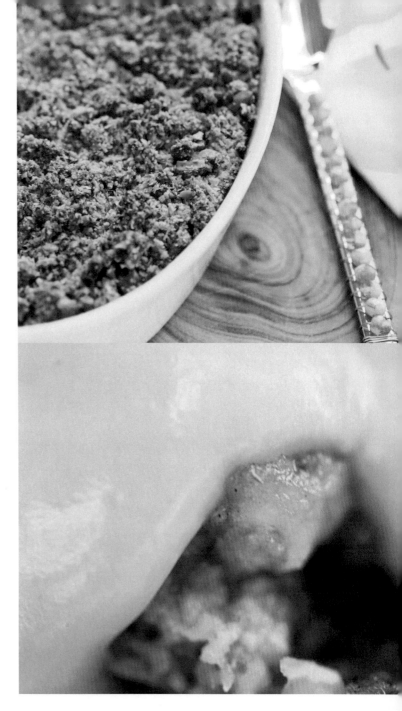

apple crumble

800 g Granny Smith apples, peeled, cubed
  and steamed (or tinned pie apple)
1 tsp ground cinnamon
¼ cup tapioca flour
½ cup almond meal (other nut meals work too)
½ cup gluten-free rolled oats, processed
  until fine
¼ cup coconut sugar
½ cup walnuts, crumbled
½ cup desiccated coconut
Pinch of fine Himalayan rock salt
40 g Nuttelex, soft but not melted
1 tbsp water

Preheat oven to 175° celcius. Place the apple in a deep casserole dish and mix the cinnamon through. Spread the apple evenly over the base of the dish - it should come up the sides of the dish about 5 cm.

In a separate bowl, combine all dry ingredients. Add the Nuttelex and water, then using your fingertips, work these wet ingredients through the dry ingredients until the mixture has moistened. Sprinkle evenly over the apple and press down gently. Bake for 35-40 minutes. Serve hot with almond custard.

There are a few different brands of gluten-free custard powder on the market. I haven't tried all of them so check the consistency of the custard and adjust with either a little more custard powder or more almond milk. Generally, I find I need to decrease the milk suggested on the packet to make a nice thick custard.

almond custard

2 tbsp gluten-free custard powder
1 ½ tbsp coconut sugar
400 ml almond milk

Put 50 ml of the almond milk in a saucepan. Add the custard powder and coconut sugar and mix until there are no lumps. Add the rest of the almond milk and stir constantly over a medium heat until the custard is thick and smooth.

Variations: Add a blended banana or mashed mango to cold custard. For something really special, scrape the vanilla beans from inside a vanilla pod and add to warm custard.

chocolate mousse

1 ripe banana, peeled and chopped
1 ripe avocado, peeled and chopped
2 tbsp honey
2 tbsp raw cacao powder
½ tsp ground cinnamon
½ tsp fine Himalayan rock salt

Place all ingredients in a high-walled bowl. Using a stick mixer, blend all ingredients until combined, thick and glossy. Spoon into bowls and serve immediately. Serves 4 small or 2 large.

Also great sprinkled with fresh seasonal berries!

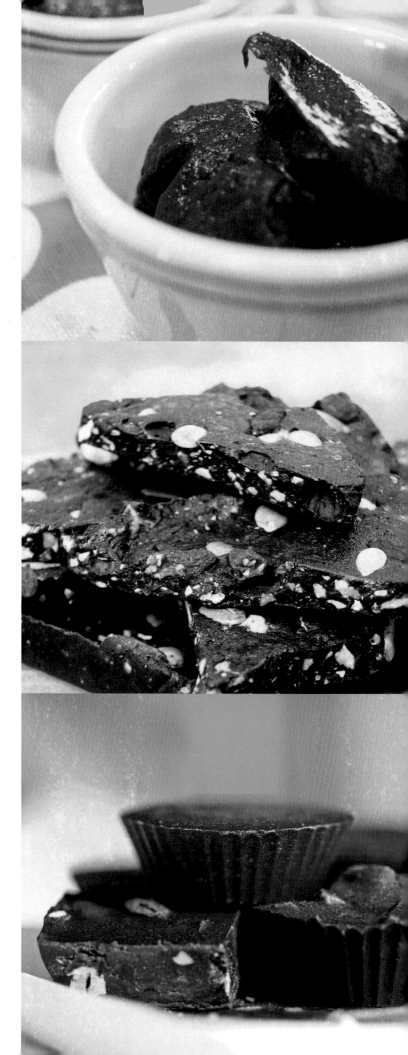

chocolate bark

140 g cacao wafers
¼ cup maple syrup
½ tsp fine Himalayan rock salt
½ tsp mixed spice
¼ cup hazelnuts, roughly chopped
¼ cup pepitas
½ cup dried goji berries and/or cranberries

Melt the cacao wafers in a bowl over a saucepan of simmering water and when melted, remove from the heat. Quickly add the maple syrup, salt, mixed spice and nuts. Stir through until combined.

Spoon the mixture into a slice tin lined with baking paper and spread out evenly with a spatula. Sprinkle pepitas and dried cranberries on the top. Place a small sheet of baking paper over the mixture and press down with the palm of your hand until the chocolate bark is flat and an even thickness. Leaving the paper on top, place in the fridge until firm. Peel paper off chocolate, break into rustic pieces and store airtight in the fridge.

Excellent quality chocolate is food for the soul, providing us with nutrients and antioxidants, feelings of relaxation and sometimes euphoria. My husband is a self-confessed chocoholic and so our family's new eating regime stifled his addiction big time! When I started making the Honey Chocolate he fell in love with me all over again and life in our house has now returned to normal.

The Chocolate Mousse is great for babies, the Chocolate Bark is a lovely festive treat and the Choc Orange Truffles make fab Easter eggs!

choc orange truffles

1 cup raw cashews
½ cup pitted dates
½ cup raisins
1 cup orange juice
1 tbsp of flaxseeds soaked in 1 tbsp of water
   for 10 mins
¾ cup raw cacao powder
1 heaped tsp orange zest
½ tsp fine Himalayan rock salt
Desiccated coconut or extra raw cacao powder
   for rolling

Soak cashews, dates and raisins in the orange juice overnight. Drain the nuts and fruit and reserve these juices. Combine all the ingredients in a food processor and blend until smooth. Add just enough of the reserved juices until the mixture is a stiff consistency. Roll spoonfuls of mixture into walnut-sized balls. To roll the ball without it sticking to your hands, rub a little coconut oil onto your palms. Then roll the ball in coconut or raw cacao powder. Freeze or refrigerate.

EASTER EGG TRUFFLES
Mould the Choc Orange Truffle mixture into egg-shaped truffles by hand (instead of balls).

honey chocolate

95 g cacao butter
35 g coconut oil
100 g honey
¾ cup raw cacao powder
2 tbsp lucuma powder
¼ tsp fine Himalayan rock salt

Melt coconut oil and cacao butter in a bowl over a saucepan of simmering water. Take off the heat and add all other ingredients, whisking together till smooth. Pour into silicone cups, chocolate moulds or a lined tray (to be cut into pieces when set). Store in the fridge.

Variation: Add your choice of nuts, dried fruit, coconut, cacao nibs or rice puffs to the mix.

HONEY CHOCOLATE ICING
For a delicious, light and creamy icing, add 3 tablespoons of thick coconut cream to the partially set chocolate. (Use the cream from the top of a cold tin of coconut cream). Whip with a stick mixer. Great as a quick, easy ganache-style cake icing.

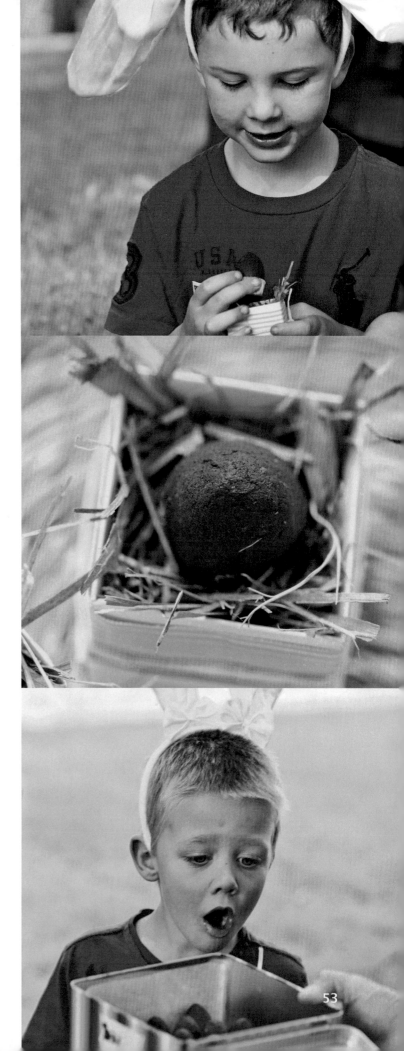

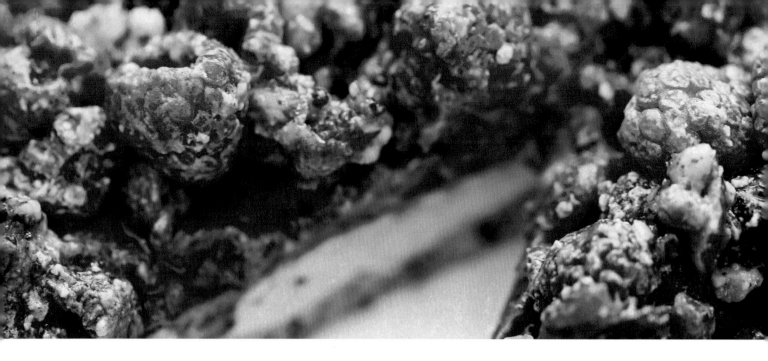

cashew, macadamia & raspberry tart

Adapted from Olivia Newton-John's 'Livwise' recipe book published by Murdoch Books.

CRUST
¼ cup desiccated coconut
2 cups macadamia nuts
½ cup pitted dates, chopped

FILLING
2 cups raw cashews (soaked in water
  overnight then drained)
Juice of 1 lemon
¼ cup maple syrup
¼ cup coconut oil, warmed
1 tsp natural vanilla essence

RASPBERRY TOPPING
2 cups raspberries, fresh or frozen
½ cup pitted dates, chopped

Lightly grease a round 22 cm spring-form cake tin. Line the base with baking paper and dust with the coconut. Put the macadamias and dates into a food processor and process until well combined. Press the mixture over the coconut into the base of the tin. To make the filling, put the cashews, lemon juice, maple syrup, coconut oil, vanilla essence and ½ cup of water into a food processor and process until smooth. Pour over the date mixture in the tin. Lightly tap the tin on the bench to remove any air bubbles. Cover with a plate and freeze for at least 2 hours or until the filling is firm. To make the topping, put the raspberries and dates in a food processor and process until smooth. Pour the topping onto the frozen tart, cover and freeze again. Remove the tart from the tin to serve.

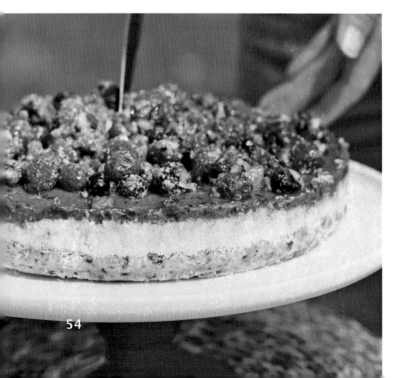

berry crumble

Adapted from Jo Whitton's Berry Nut Nougat with Raw Cacao Nibs, quirkycooking.blogspot.com.au.

100 g almonds
2 tbsp nut butter
½ cup raisins or sultanas
45 ml maple syrup
¼ cup raw cacao nibs
400 g frozen mixed berries

Process all ingredients, except the mixed berries, until almonds are well chopped. Add berries and process quickly until combined. Store in freezer. Crumble over tart before serving.

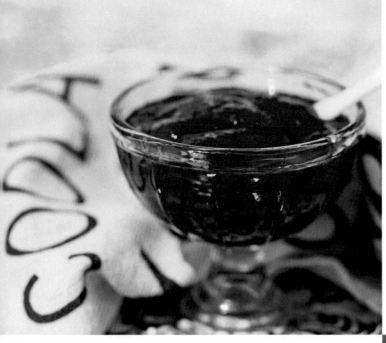

berry sorbet

2 cups frozen mixed berries
2 tbsp fresh lime juice
2 tbsp coconut sugar
1 tbsp fresh mint, chopped

Process all ingredients and serve in a glass or small bowl. You can adjust these ingredients to taste.

Very refreshing and a great palate cleanser. Also delicious as a summery dinner party dessert.

These cool treats are a hit with our kids. They love making them as much as they love eating them!

mango ice blocks

450 g ripe mango pieces, cubed
250 ml coconut cream (without additives if available)
¼ cup maple syrup
½ cup macadamia nuts, chopped (or hazelnuts)

Loosely pack mango cubes into the length of BPA-free ice block moulds. If you don't have moulds, you can use little ramekins or cups with spoons (or small wooden sticks) for the handles. Place a sprinkling of nuts on top of the mango. Mix the coconut cream and the maple syrup together then pour over the fruit and nuts. Jiggle the mixture so the coconut cream mix goes all the way down to the bottom of the mould. Place the handles into the mould and freeze until solid.

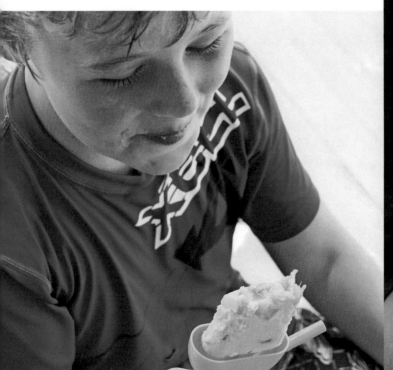

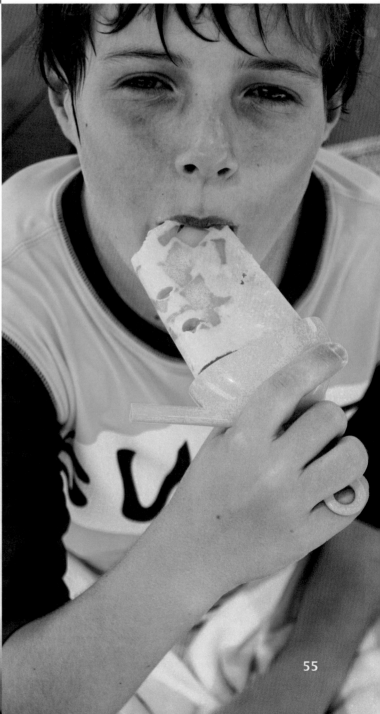

drinks

Filtered room-temperature water is what our children drink mostly from day to day, so I love offering them drinks from this section as a treat - they are also a hit at kid's birthday parties! During the day I drink water or caffeine-free rooibos tea and at night I enjoy a glass of soda water with a twist of fresh lime juice and a few drops of stevia. My daughter loves making lemonade for the family and delights in garnishing our drinks with parsley (or anything pretty) and decorating the glass rims with lemon.

watermelon slushies

2 kg approx. watermelon pieces (skin off)
  (or enough to make 6 cups of juice)
100 ml fresh lemon juice
100 ml fresh lime juice
1 tsp cayenne pepper

Process the watermelon pieces then press the mix through a strainer to collect the juice. Add this juice to all other ingredients in a large flat dish, mix and freeze. Break up pieces of the frozen watermelon mix and process until slushy.

Take martini-style glasses and dip the top edge of the glass in a plate of shallow water then spoon colourful mineral salt over the edge of the wet rim. Great salts to use are red Alaean sea salt or fine pink Himalayan rock salt. Spoon the watermelon slushies into the glasses and garnish with mint.

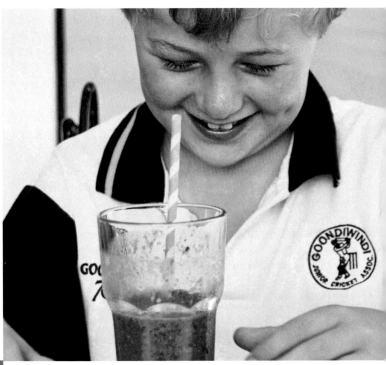

raspberry smoothies

1 frozen banana, chopped
½ cup raspberries, fresh or frozen
½ cup rice milk or alternative milk of choice
2 tsp honey (optional)
1 tbsp LSA (ground linseeds, sunflower seeds
  and almonds)

Combine all ingredients in a food processor and blend until smooth.

If using really ripe frozen bananas, you'll probably find you don't need to include the honey. You can also vary the kinds of berries used in this recipe.

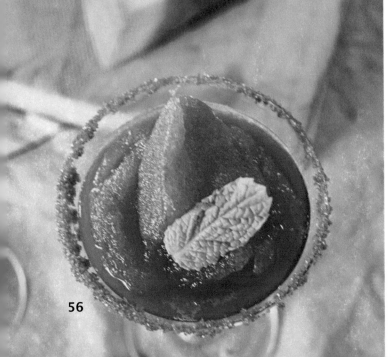

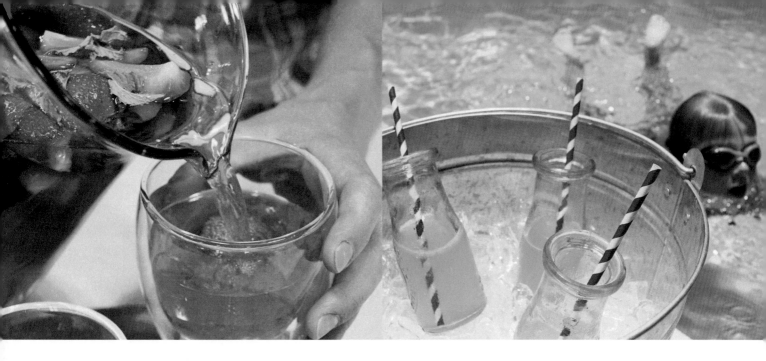

roseberry iced tea

4 cups rosehip tea
500 ml apple juice (freshly juiced if possible)
250 ml sparkling mineral water
1 cup mixed fresh berries, chopped
¼ cup fresh mint, chopped
Ice cubes

Follow the packet instructions for making 4 cups of tea. When cool, place the tea in a large glass jug and add all the remaining ingredients. Mix well and serve.

Look for the best quality rosehip tea you can find. Be mindful that many popular herbal teas contain inferior tea leaves and additives. Choose loose leaf tea where possible or tea in unbleached tea bags.

lemonade

50 ml fresh lemon juice (bush lemons
  are lovely if you can find them)
2 tsp maple syrup
Soda water to taste
Ice cubes

Mix all ingredients and stir. Use as much soda water as you like to satisfy your taste. Serves 1.

This recipe has been used by our kids to raise money for their school. They love it, especially because they can make it on their own. It's also a great source of vitamin C.

Enjoy all these refreshing drinks on a warm day!

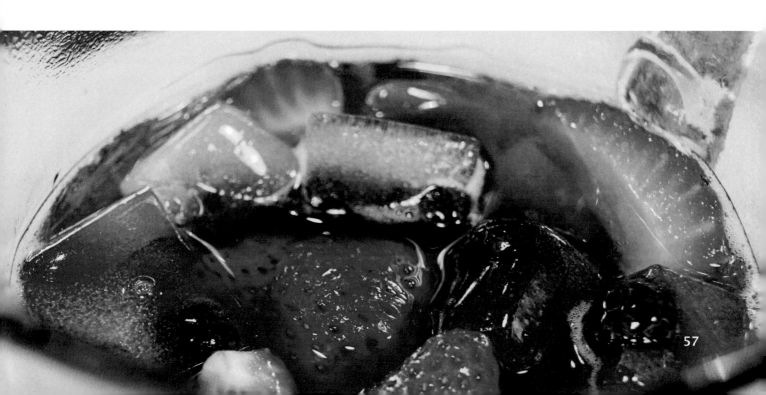

57

ConDimEnts

I am such a condiment person. I enjoy relishes, sauces and dressings with my meats and salads. The only thing is, I have to make them all myself as commercial relishes and sauces give me stomach aches and reflux. I don't mind because I can really taste the wholefood flavours in homemade condiments; they aren't masked with additives or excess sugar and salt. Try the Raisin Relish for a fresh zing with a summer salad or enjoy the authentic flavour of the Caper and Dill Sauce with a piece of grilled fish.

onion jam

700 g brown onion
½ cup extra-virgin olive oil
1 large bay leaf
1 tbsp mixed dried herbs
1 small sprig fresh rosemary
1 tsp fine Himalayan rock salt

Peel and chop onions finely. In a heavy-based saucepan over a high heat, bring all ingredients to the boil and then turn the heat to low. With the lid on simmer for 30-40 minutes, stirring intermittently or until soft and jam-like. Place in an appropriate container and seal. Keeps in the fridge for 4-5 days.

I keep this jam on hand as it's a great base for many dishes. I blend a portion and add to sauces, gravies, soups and dips to thicken and enhance flavour. Also delicious on crackers or fresh bread.

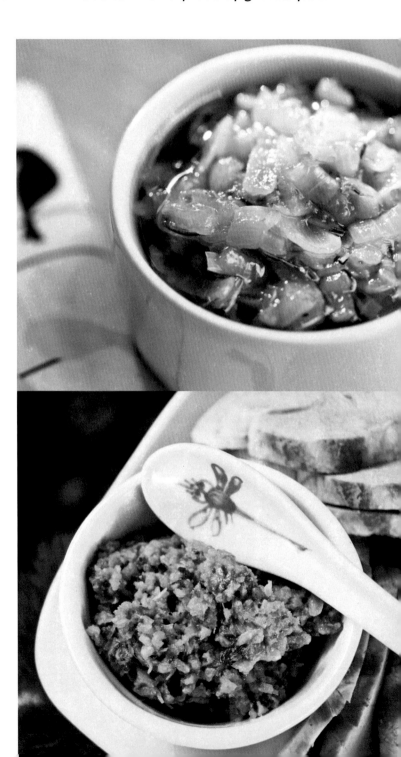

raisin relish

25 g onion, roughly chopped
150 g celery, roughly chopped
40 g raisins
1 tbsp apple cider vinegar
1 tsp extra-virgin olive oil
¼ tsp mixed spice
Fine Himalayan rock salt to taste
Cracked black pepper

Combine all ingredients in a food processor and process until finely chopped and amalgamated. Best eaten the day after it's made. Serve with cold meats or as a spread on a salad sandwich.

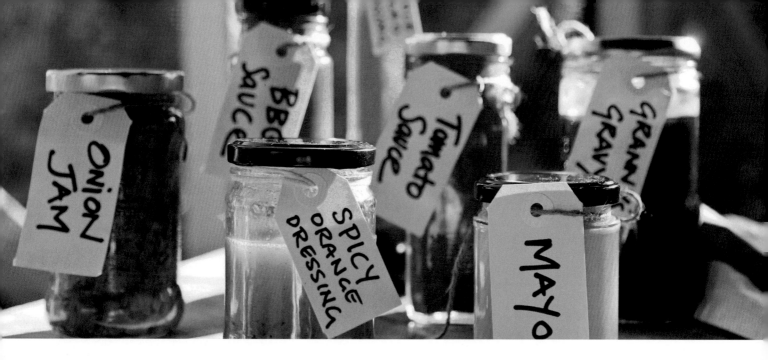

tomato sauce

200 g onion, peeled and chopped
2 tbsp extra-virgin olive oil
400 g tin diced tomatoes
1 tbsp additive-free tomato paste
1 tbsp honey
½ tsp dried chilli flakes (optional)
1 tbsp fresh mixed herbs, chopped
1 tsp fine Himalayan rock salt

Sauté onion in oil until soft and translucent. Add all other ingredients and simmer until sauce has reduced a little. Blend all ingredients until smooth. Store covered in fridge for up to 4 days. Can be frozen.

bbq sauce

Use the same recipe as the Tomato Sauce above, except add 3 tablespoons of Braggs All Purpose Seasoning and ½ teaspoon of garam masala.

meat stock

When cooking steak, lamb chops, chicken pieces, pork chops etc. reserve all the juices. If there is no juice left over, deglaze the pan with some water and scrape solid particles and juice into a freezer-proof container (excluding any burnt pieces). Skim off any excess fat. Freeze approximately 100 ml portions to use in place of stock cubes.

mayonnaise

Adapted from a cleangreensimple.com recipe.

½ cup Azalea 100% pure grapeseed oil
¼ cup gluten-free soy milk
½ tsp fine Himalayan rock salt
2 tsp apple cider vinegar
2 tsp maple syrup

In a small food processor, whip oil and milk until well combined and thickened. This takes about 3-4 minutes. Add half the vinegar and syrup then process until thick again. Add remaining vinegar and salt then process until well combined. Makes approximately 1 cup of mayonnaise.

Garlic aioli variation:
Add 1-2 crushed garlic cloves to final mix.

Herbed variation for potato salad:
Add a level tablespoon each, of chopped parsley, peppery rocket and mint.

granny's gravy

100 ml meat stock
1 ½ cups water
1 heaped tbsp cornflour mixed in 1 tbsp water
1 tsp honey
2 tsp fine Himalayan rock salt (or to taste)

Heat and stir all ingredients in a saucepan until combined and gravy has thickened. Adjust to preferred consistency with water or alternatively add a little more cornflour and water.

spicy orange dressing

1 ½ tbsp orange juice
½ tbsp fresh lemon juice
2 ½ tbsp extra-virgin olive oil
1 garlic clove, crushed
Fine Himalayan rock salt to taste
Cracked black pepper

In a jar with lid on, shake all ingredients together until well combined. Pour over salad and toss.

Enjoy with the Quinoa & Cranberry Chicken Salad (see page 29).

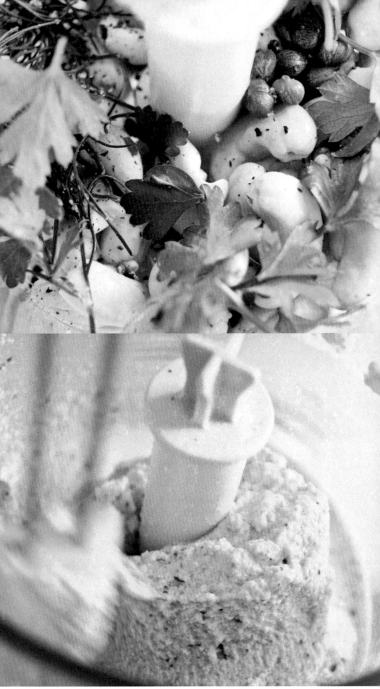

caper & dill sauce

½ cup raw cashews, soaked
1 tsp capers, drained and rinsed
1 tsp fresh dill
1 tsp fresh parsley
½ garlic clove, crushed (or to taste)
Juice of ½ a lemon
Fine Himalayan rock salt to taste
Cracked black pepper

Soak the cashews in warm water for at least 2 hours, preferably overnight, then purée with enough of the soaking water to make a thick sauce. Add the rest of the ingredients and blend until smooth. For a thinner sauce, add more soaking water.

This sauce is a lovely, refreshing accompaniment to the Barra Fish Fingers (see page 33).

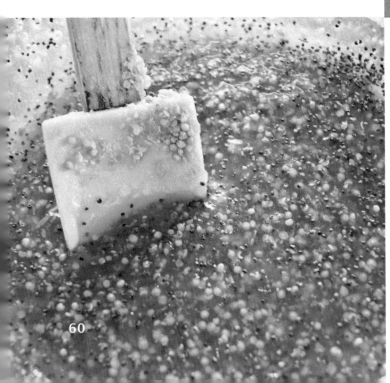

honey mustard dressing

2 tbsp yellow mustard seeds, roughly ground in a mortar and pestle
1 tbsp poppy seeds
2 tbsp fresh lemon juice
4 tbsp honey
½ tsp fine Himalayan rock salt

Combine all ingredients together.

Great with the Baby Spinach & Pumpkin Salad (see page 28).

Healthy Home

Guided by information I have gathered over the years pertaining to possible Scleroderma causes, along with changes to my diet, I have adopted the relevant practices listed below and eliminated certain products from our home to reduce our exposure to chemicals. Eliminating these types of products has helped alleviate symptoms I used to experience on a daily basis, such as headaches, itchy skin and heartburn.

Reducing the chemical load in our home has freed up our senses to enjoy all the pure and natural elements in our environment.

- Eliminate as many cleaning chemicals from your home as possible, especially antibacterial and bleach products.
- Use vinegar and bicarb soda for cleaning.
- Fragrance your home with essential oils, fresh herbs and flowers.
- Find healthier, chemical-free alternatives for beauty products and toiletries.
- Limit your exposure to new plastic products.
- Use BPA-free babies bottles and soothers.
- Lather your children's hair with conditioner and comb out lice rather than using chemicals.
- Always wash new clothes, soft furnishings and bedding before use.
- Use unscented washing powder.
- When purchasing fabric for your body and home, choose natural fibres.
- Grow or buy organic food when possible.
- If you can eat eggs and keep your own chooks, be mindful of how much grain/gluten they eat.
- If your body can tolerate dairy products, milk your own goat or cow if possible.

- Always read the labels on your food and avoid additives and preservatives.
- Use glass or ceramic containers to store food and avoid using plastic food wrap.
- Use a water filter and avoid buying water in plastic throwaway bottles.
- Manually remove cobwebs from your home rather than spraying spiders with chemicals.
- Use a fly swatter or screen your house from flies and insects.
- Research and use safer alternatives to estapols and enamel paints.
- Reduce exposure to electromagnetic energy e.g. mobile phones, TVs and computers.
- If you live near a rock quarry or coal mine, seal your house well and create effective buffer zones using plants and trees to protect your home and family from the dust.
- Any form of reduction is a good thing, so do what is practical and give yourself time to eliminate contaminants from your home.

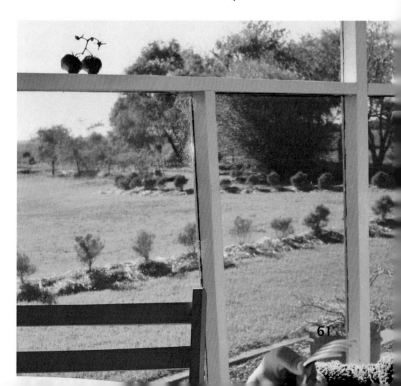

FooD For ThouGht

I've been blown away by the feeling of wellness that has come over me since I stopped eating particular foods. This feeling seems to translate into a positive energy that changes the world around me.

Sounds a little corny I know but it's true. I'm still getting used to the wonderful experiences this feeling has brought into my life. I now have a new appreciation for the power of food!

I'd love to share some other insights with you that I've discovered whilst on my healing journey:

Food prepared and served with love, nourishes and heals the body, mind and spirit.

- Saying grace or thanks before a meal creates an uplifting energy around the table.
- Positive words and thoughts are healing, as proven by Dr Masaru Emoto's ground-breaking research and water crystal photography.
- Food has the potential to bring people, who normally don't get along, together for special occasions and inevitably there is laughter!
- Using our best china makes every meal a celebration and helps us feel worthy.
- Eating and appreciating good quality food in good company helps us feel happy.
- Understanding which emotions affect which organs of the body helps us heal.
- Healing is easier and more effective when we eat foods in season, as nature intended.
- Our bodies don't lie - listening to what they're saying before they have to shout is wise.
- The truth heals and can inspire us to act.
- Exercising makes life comfortable and joyful.
- Trust your intuition and enjoy an easier life!

I have come to realise it was when I chose to be really happy and accept myself that I truly began to heal. This was a defining moment which inspired me to set out alone to write a book of recipes that I hoped would help others feel good. However 'Friendship Food' would not have evolved and be the book that it is, if I had continued to plug along by myself without the help of my friends. Working with the girls and in particular, very closely with Jules on formatting this book, has changed my life as I now consciously think, write, act and speak more optimistically.

'Friendship Food' has been an optimistic leap of faith itself in many ways. It's our first homegrown attempt to create and self-publish a book and although we have lots to learn, we offer you a real snapshot of our lives in the spirit of encouraging other friends to join forces to fulfill their dreams!

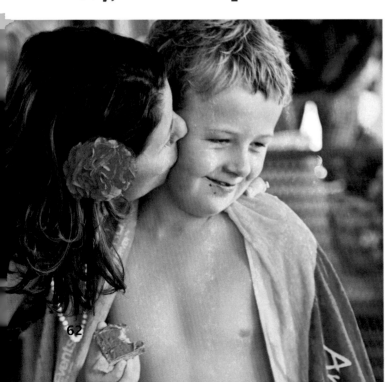

Thank You

A year ago Kate asked me 'Flick, what's happening with the book?' I remarked to her that it was making progress at a snail's pace as I was readjusting to life as a mother of four. In her true pragmatic, get-things-done style, Kate said 'you've had your baby, back to it, chop, chop' and with that she offered to help by test-cooking all the recipes. Kate mentioned to her sister Jules that I needed a photographer. Jules happily took on this role and so the production of the book fired ahead.

When Jules started sending through those first gorgeous pictures of the food, I realised very emotionally that my dream was becoming a reality. Some months later Kylie, my Salt of Life business partner and good friend, joined us for what has become a pivotal year. It has been a joy to work and grow alongside these three talented women.

'Friendship Food' has grown because we believe that great things in life begin with great relationships - whether it is with your body, food, family, the environment, or of course your friends.

To Kate, Jules and Kylie, thank you dearly. Your generosity and unconditional faith in me is very humbling. With your input, creating this book has become so much more than producing a book of recipes. It has become an inspiring part of my healing journey and it has helped me realise our dreams can come true when we feel good!

My family, you are the single greatest achievement of my life. Trev you are the kindest, most amazing husband and father. You once told me that I saved you. I think together with Tom, Mimi, George and Maggie, you have all saved me from myself. Thank you, my heart feels full of love and gratitude. As a parent I am honoured that some universal power sent the four of you to us with the responsibility to shape you into the beautiful souls you have the potential to be. I love helping you prepare for your future and even if I seem a little busy sometimes, I am always thinking of ways to guide you and advise you on choosing the safest, happiest journey through this wonderful life we are gifted with.

Mum and Dad thank you for your unconditional love. I feel it always. Let's happily make the most of the rest of our days - there's no time to waste. Melissa and Jack thanks for the happy childhood memories, the shoulders to cry on and the lives and families we now share. As siblings, you're alright you know!

Many people in this world have inspired me for many reasons. Below is my list of food inspirers. My knowledge base has been enhanced by their experiences and their delicious and nutritious food. Thanks to Barbara Cousins, Teresa Cutter, Tania Hubbard, Therese and Miranda Kerr, Erin McKenna, Olivia Newton-John, Jamie Oliver, Cyndi O'Meara, Janella Purcell and Jo Whitton.

To all those qualified authors of good nutrition and health information, thank you. The more I learn, the more I realise I have yet to learn. Finally, thank *you* for taking the time to read my story. I'd love it to help at least one person enjoy greater health and happiness - maybe that person is you?

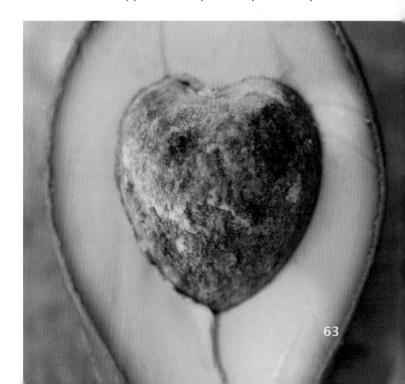

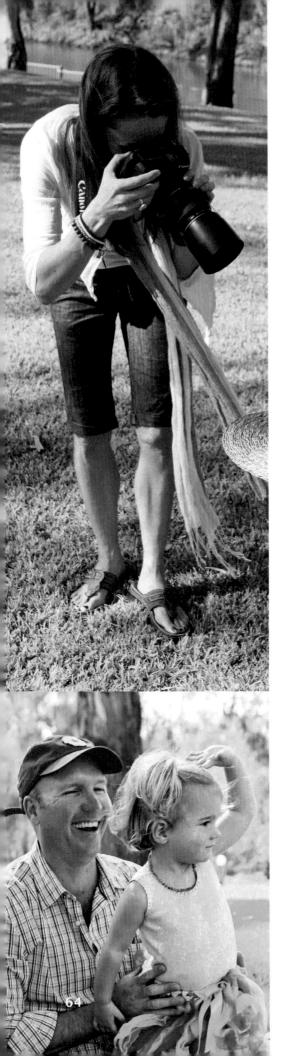

InDex

A

Activated nuts & seeds 16
Alcohol 6, 8, 9, 13, 18, 37
Allergy 6
Almond milk 16
Antibiotics 6
Apple cider vinegar 16
Arrowroot 16
Arsenic 12
Arthritis 9, 14
Asthma 6, 19
Autoimmunity / Autoimmune
      disorder 3, 4, 6, 9, 14

B

Baking powder 16
Barley 6
Besan flour 16
Braggs All Purpose Seasoning 17
Breads & Loaves 5, 40-43
Breakfast 5, 20-23
Buckwheat flour 17

C

Cacao
      bean 17
      butter 17
      nibs 17
      raw powder 17
      wafers 17
Cakes, Bars & Biscuits 5, 44-49
Cancer 8,17
Candidiasis 6, 14
Cane sugar 7
Cardiovascular disease 8
Casein 6
Chemicals 6, 12, 13, 17, 19, 61
Chia seeds 17
Cigarettes 13
Coconut
      oil / butter 17
      sugar 17
Coeliac disease 6, 18
Condiments 5, 58-60
Connective tissue 9
Cornflour 17
Cow's milk 10, 19, 61
Cravings 6, 14, 17

D

'Dirty Dozen' 12
Dairy 6, 7, 14
Desserts & Sweet Treats 5, 50-55
Diabetes 6, 8, 9, 17, 18
Disease 3, 8, 9
Drinks 5, 56, 57

E

Eggs 6, 61
Elimination diet 3, 7, 14
Extra-virgin olive oil 17

F

Flaxseeds 18
Food intolerance 4, 6
'Friendship Food' 2, 3, 62, 63, 79
Fruit 7, 20
Fungal yeast, 6 *also see*
      Candidiasis 6, 14

G

Glucose 6, 7
Gluten 6, 7, 14
Gluten-free products 18
Glycaemic Index 6, 7
Grave's disease 9

H

Hashimoto's disease 9
Honey 18

I

Immune system 6, 7, 9, 12, 17
Infections, chest and viral 7
Inflammation 7
Ingredients 16-19
Insulin 6, 9
Irritable Bowel Syndrome 6

J

K

L

Lactose 6, 16, 19
Libido 14
Lipids 6
Lucuma powder 18
Lupus 9

M

Macadamia oil 18
Main Meals 5, 30-35
Maple syrup 18
Measuring equipment 15
Mental clarity 14
Miscarriage 12, 13
Multiple Sclerosis 9

N

Nibbles, Dips & Crackers 5, 36-39
Nut butters 18
Nuttelex 18

O

Obesity 8
Oral contraception 6

P

Pancreas 7
Pantry 15, 16
Persistent Organic Pollutants 12
Pizza 42, 43
Polenta 18
Pomegranate molasses 18
Psoriasis 14

Q

Quinoa 18, 29, 40, 41

R

Refined sugar 6,7,13,14,17,18,19
Rheumatoid Arthritis 9
Rice
    crumbs 18
    milk 19
Rye 6

S

Salads & Light Meals 5, 26-29
Salt 19
Scleroderma 3, 9, 12, 13, 14, 61
Self-esteem 13, 14,

Sjogren's syndrome 9
Sodium bicarbonate 16, 61
Soups 5, 24, 25
Soy products 19
Stevia 19
Subcutaneous calcinosis 14
Sugar 6, 7, 9, 14, 17, 18, 19
Sulphite-free dried fruit 19
Symptoms
    bloating 6, 7, 14
    breath / body odour 6, 14
    colds 6
    coughing / congestion 10
    cramps 6, 7, 14
    diarrhoea 6, 14
    headaches 14, 61
    heartburn 14, 46, 61
    mood swings 6
    mouth ulcers 6
    nausea 6, 7
    plantar warts 6
    post nasal drip 6
    premenstrual tension 14
    puffy hands / feet 13, 14
    restless legs 14
    sinus 6
    skin problems 6
    sore joints 9, 14
    stress 8, 12, 14, 17
    thrush 6, 7
    tiredness 14
    vomiting 7
    wind 6, 7, 14

T

Tahini 19
Tamari 19
Tapioca flour 19
Tinned foods 19

U

V

Vegetable 7, 8, 9, 37
Vinegar 16, 61

W

Wheat 6, 14, 30

X

Xanthan gum 19

Y

Yeast 6, 7, 14

Z

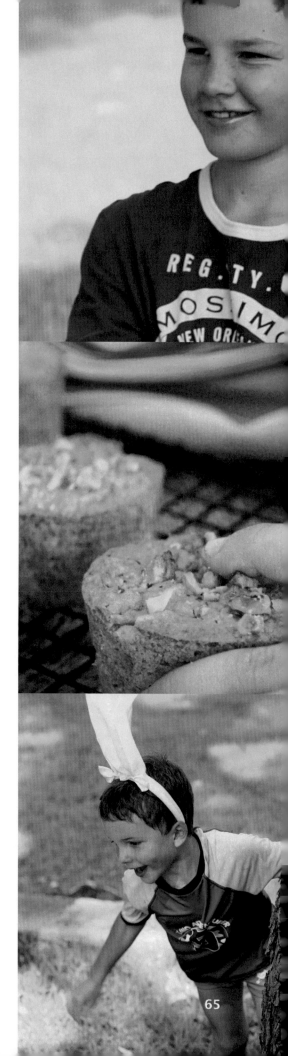

References

Over the past five years I have read some very interesting information pertaining to food, diet and health and I have made some informative and empowering discoveries. A gigantic THANK YOU to all the people and organisations behind the websites below. Key posts on these sites have enriched my life with beneficial information which has helped me heal and create this book.

allergicliving.com
bodyandsoul.com.au
changinghabits.com.au
cleangreensimple.com
epa.nsw.gov.au
fedup.com.au
foodintolerances.com.au
foodintol.com
glucoseintolerantdiet.com
glutenfreecooking.about.com
haveyougottheguts.com
healthguidance.org
hemocode.com
keeperofthehome.org
koraorganics.com
livestrong.com
masaru-emoto.net
medicinenet.com
mbm.net.au

naturalhealthclinic.com.au
natural-health-information-centre.com
newscientist.com
oprah.com
powersuperfoods.com
quirkycooking.blogspot.com.au
sallyjoseph.com.au
scleroderma.org.au
sclerodermaaustralia.com.au
taniaspantry.com
thehealthychef.com
thenourishedlife.com.au
thewellnesswarrior.com.au
thewholisticingredient.com
who.int
wikipedia.org

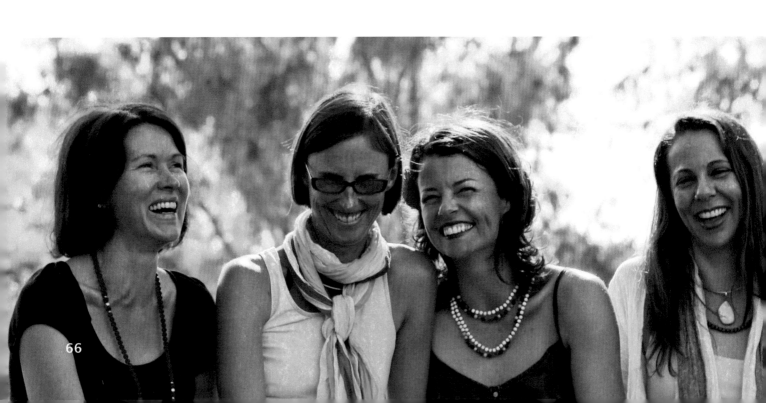

Notes

The greatest sweetener
of human life is friendship.

Joseph Addison (1672-1719)

Happiness is homemade.

Anon

**What is done in love
is done well!**

Vincent Van Gogh (1853-1890)

**One cannot think well, love well, sleep well,
if one has not dined well.**

Virginia Woolf (1882-1941)

**Let food be your medicine and
medicine be your food.**

Hippocrates (c.460-c.370 BC)

I love people who make me laugh.
I honestly think it's the thing I like most, to laugh.
It cures a multitude of ills.

Audrey Hepburn (1929-1993)

**Laughter is brightest
in the place where the food is.**

Irish Proverb

If you have good thoughts,
they will shine out of your face like sunbeams
and you will always look lovely.

Roald Dahl (1916-1990)

**Optimism is the faith
that leads to achievement.**

Helen Keller (1880-1968)

**Be who you were created to be
and you will set the world on fire.**

St Catherine of Sienna (1347-1380)

**Nothing is impossible,
the word itself says 'I'm possible'.**

Audrey Hepburn (1929-1993)

I am still learning.

Michelangelo at age 87 (1475-1564)

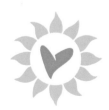

Share | Enjoy | Nourish | Thrive

friendshipfood.com.au

Printed in the United States
By Bookmasters